Toolkit for Wellness

Master Your Health and Stress Response for Life

Deidre Edwards

ISBN: 978-1518692765

Typeset by Angelique Mroczka

Printed in the United States of America

This book is dedicated to the memory of my mother who planted the seeds of personal responsibility and a keen interest in improving health through nutrition.

CONTENTS

BONUS MATERIALS

Thank you for purchasing *Toolkit for Wellness*.

As a thank gift to make your personal journey to life-long health more fun and to guarantee your success at easily applying small changes, here is a link for you to access ALL of the Bonus Materials that are mentioned throughout *Toolkit for Wellness*.

GO TO THE LINK BELOW:

https://booklaunch.io/deidre/toolkit-for-wellness

Your Bonus Materials include:

- Easy Tweaks to Living Better
- Easy Tweaks Habit Tracker
- Easy Tweaks for Starting an Exercise Plan
- Perfect Plate Template

All of your Bonus Materials are downloadable and printable for your easy access and inspiration.

Follow the effortless steps outlined in *Toolkit for Wellness* to start your habit and wellness transformation today!

As you will learn soon, attempting massive habit changes is a daunting task when attempted the wrong way. *Toolkit for Wellness* will put the tools and the know-how into your hands and mind that will transform your ability to exact great changes to your health and wellness through very doable, repeatable, daily steps that require no will power!

GO HERE TO GET YOUR BONUS MATERIALS:

https://booklaunch.io/deidre/toolkit-for-wellness

FOREWORD

Nature or nurture? A little of both I guess. Maybe, I am a natural life-long learner, as seen in my mid-life return to college to become an RN; or maybe, I became a lifelong learner due to my nearly 20 year background as a National Board Certified Teacher in Career and Technical Education, wherein we impart and demonstrate a love of life-long learning to our students.

In any case, learning is a fascination to me and literally defines my being alive because growing *is* life. Nothing in nature just is. Everything is growing, except maybe for rocks; but I am not a rock!

I am especially a seeker and giver of inspiration. In so doing, four quotes have substantially spurred me forward to action.

> "What would you do if you weren't afraid?"
> —Spencer Johnson, *Who Moved My Cheese?*

This first one made me realize how silly my fear of singing solos was. "If I was not afraid, I would sing a solo at church." Really? I already was singing in several choirs, beaming with each song's meaning. Where was my faith in terms of singing a solo? Well, I put myself out there when the invitation was made to try out for a solo, and BAM. One, two, three solos under my belt!

> "It doesn't matter if you're trying to start a business, lose weight, write a book, or achieve any number of goals... who you are, what you have, and what you know *right now* is good enough to get going."

—James Clear, newsletter, "Successful People Start Before They Feel Ready." November 2013

Then, armed with the successful application of the first quote, I really wanted to share the results of my constant studies about nutrition and wellness. I kept reading from favorite on-line authors, such as James Clear, in his research about habit formation and daily application of any skill—which leads to the third quote—and I kept thinking about starting my own blog. There always seemed to be a huge running up to the start and then stopping, only to step back to run up to the start again and again. I seemed to be waiting for everything to be perfect and in place before I started. And yet, individuals were always coming up to me for dietary advice. They wanted me to write about it!

"Much good that might have been achieved in the world is lost through hesitation, faltering, wavering, vacillating, or just not sticking with it."
—William J. Bennett, *Book of Virtues*

Enter Bennett's quote about hesitation. I knew that other people had directly benefited by applying information I shared with them; who was *not* improving their health because I had *not* started my blog or my teaching of *Designed for Health* classes? Clearly there was a mission! "Here am I Lord, send me!"

"Every sustained action, no matter how small, will bring results."
—Michal Stawicki, *Master Your Time in 10 Minutes a Day*

With my head full of ideas and a renewed thirst for knowledge, there was so much I wanted to do to improve my own self first, and then to share what worked with others, but where to start? The ultimate goal seemed too daunting at times until my eyes were opened to the mechanics of changing habits and reaching goals. I learned how to implement small changes over time and discovered that my consistent efforts did, indeed, yield great results.

Where are you in your life's journey? Looking for direction? Inspiration? An answer about healthful eating that finally makes sense? A way that spurs you on to wellness that does not require sheer willpower?

I hope that something I share with you in this book may become your inspiration and help you to take action, in some aspect, of your improved wellness. What are you afraid of? Why are you hesitating? There is a good way to start change in your life and there is a bad way. I want to show you the way that is totally doable and the one that will give you the results you want!

DISCLAIMER

The information shared and expressed in this book is not intended to replace a relationship with a qualified health care provider. This book is about empowering people through the exploration of publicly available resource information about human anatomy and physiology, and how different foods affect the human body.

Readers should seek the advice of their qualified health care providers with any questions about their medical conditions or health status before attempting any dietary, exercise, or lifestyle changes. I am not responsible for any adverse results that may ensue from the reader's application of any information shared in this book.

I write about changes to habits, diet, stress response, and exercise applied in my own life and in others I have seen. Personal responses and results are always unique. This is especially important if you have preexisting health concerns. Coordinating with your health care provider first is always best.

Mention of specific individuals, authorities, companies, or organizations does not imply an endorsement by this author or the publisher. Except for my connection as an affiliate for Self-Publishing School, this author received no compensation or incentive to promote the companies, products, or organizations mentioned in this book.

INTRODUCTION

This *Toolkit for Wellness* was written for the confused and conflicted among us who have been bombarded with so many opposing messages about what to eat, how to approach improved health, and how to exercise, that they feel overwhelmed and unable to take a confident first step to improving their and their family's health.

This book is for you if these statements and questions sound all too familiar:

- I give up! The government and experts are always changing their minds on what we should be eating.

- Surely, choosing a healthy diet can be easier. Who am I to believe?

- Yo-yo dieting describes my past experiences. I am carrying more weight and feel worse than ever. Help!

- Do I really know how my body responds to different foods? Is that even important?

- Is food related to how I think and solve problems?

- Is there a cure to my "foggy brain"?

- Am I nourishing my family for optimal health?

- Can I feel better by eating differently?

- Is my bad sleeping affecting my weight, and what can I do about it?

- Stress is my middle name!

This book is definitely **not** for you if you embrace the following thoughts:

- I like what I am eating and the way I live. I just want to take a pill to fix my ailments.

- No worries, modern Western medicine and the pharmaceuticals have my back.

- If my food doesn't come prepackaged and prepared, it's not going into my mouth.

- All those unpronounceable words on my packaged food are okay because the government regulates all that stuff. It's safe for me.

- That afternoon slump is normal! Some caffeine and a honey bun, and I am raring to go!

What this book *will* do for you:

- You will become empowered. By using these tools and 'tweaks' to everyday habits, you will be well along the path to an actual reinvention and transformation of your health.

- You will learn that change is **not** a matter of sheer will power, but comes through implementation of small, painless, daily 'tweaks' to habits we already have. I'll show you how.

- You will feel better and rediscover the healthier 'you' that may have lain dormant for years under the results of layers of misinformation about food and exercise.

- You will learn about several toxic foods that have been undermining your wellbeing and how to avoid them.

- You will never be hungry! Hunger is never the way to weight loss or improved health.

- You will learn and practice how to stop the stress reaction RIGHT NOW!

- You will learn tricks to eating out and for celebrations that will support your efforts to eating better.

- You will come to the amazing truth that the answer to our increasing health crises of obesity, diabetes, auto-immune diseases, and inflammatory complications has been hidden in plain sight.

- You will discover the tools already at your disposal to regain a positive control over your mental and physical wellness. No further purchases necessary.

- You will be liberated from the daily hype, from pharmaceuticals, and mega food conglomerates with their minions who carefully point you toward a life-long dependence on their products. You will be able to understand and follow the money trail that has led to the colossal duping of Americans.

- You will marvel at how easily you will feel better mentally, physically, and spiritually.

With my background in Nursing Home Administration, nursing, and teaching as a National Board Certified Teacher in Career and Technical Education in high school Health Sciences for nearly 20 years, I have developed a passion for showing others how to better themselves through knowledge and learning.

Really learning something means there will be a resultant change in behavior because of what was learned. Early on, we all learned the meaning of "HOT" and we no longer put our curious little fingers near hot things. No change in behavior? No learning.

Whether it's issues with energy levels, weight, too many ailments, or the effects of stress, your sense of dissatisfaction with your current state of wellness is **not** to be viewed as a judgment on your efforts or of your own self. It's just a wake-up call and awareness on your part there *must* be a better way, a natural way, which does not seem so foreign to your body to work. You are most assuredly right!

Bravo! You have just taken the first step to improved results by holding this book and starting on a journey you can implement right away to feel and look better. You will gain the confidence that comes from making positive choices for yourself that are doable and repeatable. And, you will be laying the ground work for future improvements for your wellness.

This book represents a sort of 'call to arms' because I know we **can** change how we look, act, think, and feel through improved food choices, stress response modification, mindset shifts, better sleep, and consistent exercise. I have experienced this myself and have seen it in the participants who attend my *Designed for Health Seminars*. In teaching my seminars, one goal was always foremost in my mind: Giving my *Designed for Health* participants tools they can immediately and easily start using on their positive journey to improved wellness.

My goal for you, the reader, is the same. Here is a toolkit for you to feel better, look better, and live better. Many of the tools you already have, we are just going to develop them to their fullest. You are worth it! You will be fully equipped to face the future as a new and better you. Your improved health and your action plans are just a few pages away. Let's get started by unpacking that toolkit.

Volumes have been written on every topic covered in your *Toolkit for Wellness*. I may even follow up this book with others that amplify certain ideas and tips presented here. But my goal is to try to synthesize a lot of information into a cohesive single reference. I hope you enjoy having this easy-to-understand resource at your fingertips for referral.

Each section will end with a brief summary called, "Take Away Thoughts," and "Take Away Actions," meaning what ideas you should be taking away with you as a review and what actions you can immediately implement for improvement.

OUR TOOLKIT IS ABOUT WELLNESS

What Is Wellness?

We spent the first week of nursing school exploring the concept of wellness. What is it? Lack of disease? Perfect weight? What is a perfect weight, and can someone who is overweight be considered well? But people who were well physically could be very unwell mentally or spiritually. Stuff for the philosophers, perhaps.

We settled on the concept of a "wellness continuum," which is like the art class exercise of taking pure black on one side of the canvas and gradually turning it into white on the other side by using more and more white paint and decreasing the black. Our health status moves back and forth on this black-to-gray-to-white scale.

Certainly, we have to consider the wellness trifecta of an inner-relationship with all aspects of wellness: mental, physical, and emotional or spiritual. Whether you visualize three circles intersecting and overlapping, or you think more in terms of a triangle, it is easy to see how all aspects of wellness relate to each other.

We will be looking at how the body maintains its balance, which is achieved through a process called homeostasis. This process is good for balancing blood sugar, regulating internal temperature, and a host of other vital balancing acts, but it can work to our detriment if we try to really rock the boat with major habit changes.

The body likes status quo. Stability is energy efficient. Auto-pilot allows the body to glide along, not expending its limited resources for dispensing strong willpower to carry out big changes. Oh sure, every January, people from around the world feel compelled to clean up their acts: Eat better, exercise more, and start all kinds of grandiose habits. Trouble is, probably before the month is out, most of us have resumed gliding along on auto-pilot as our bodies protect that precious set-point.

So is change even possible? Certainly! As we "unwrap" your *Toolkit for Wellness*, we will be learning how to successfully implement change in our lives with relative ease! But first, I would like to share some targets for our efforts to higher levels of wellness.

Did you know that just about every disease known to mankind has roots in one particularly nasty, but totally natural body response to invaders? Inflammation. From A-Z, virtually all diseases have a causative inflammatory factor. "Gee, if we could just limit the causes of the inflammatory response we could cut down on disease!" Well, hello, we can do just that! Control *starting* inflammation by eating the right foods, and you will control one of the first dominoes from ever falling over toward disease! Tools for reversing the inflammation are already in place and will be at your fingertips. You are really in control of this.

Secondly, cutting down on physically inflaming agents will lead us to calming down inflaming factors that vex our minds and spirits. I will be addressing that right away.

Again, you are very actively in control of this as well. With consistent application of the methods shared in this book, you can achieve dramatic results for yourself.

Thirdly, when speaking of wellness, one cannot escape exercise. I tend to eschew most forms of official exercise such as going to a gym. Being active? Yes, I am definitely active and I want to do everything to stay that way. But contrary to our normal way of thinking, more exercise is not necessarily the answer. The research that has led me to understand a wiser application of body energies, along with a much deeper understanding of habit formation, have really transformed how I look at, and do, exercise. I have also learned how to avoid using sheer will power to keep moving. I can't wait to show you how.

Take Away Thoughts:

- "Wellness" is a word/concept we normally do not try to define; we think that we all know what it means.

Take Away Actions:

- It would be a revealing exercise to ask everyone around the table tonight what they considered wellness was for them. You just might learn come un-voiced concerns and the conversation would get the ball rolling on personal goals, needs, and an opportunity for a group effort.

THE MOST IMPORTANT TOOL

What's the Most Important Tool?

"Nothing exists without first being created, and in your life,
that creation begins in your mind."
—Michal Stawicki, *Mastering Your Time in 10 Minutes a Day*

We all have one!

Here's the thing. There is no escaping the truth that everything, but everything, revolves around the engagement of our brains. Eating right, being a better person, starting a new habit, taking the dog for a walk, helping our children with their homework. It all starts with a thought.

Wellness, like anything else, is a brain game, so to speak. Whether we talk about mental, physical, or spiritual health, our success totally depends upon thinking. Attitudes reflect a thought process. Happiness is a thought process. Success, at anything, starts with a thought. A belief in that thought, a visualization of that thought, a commitment to acting on that thought, and a steady application of that thought. Thinking positive things, and choosing to apply those positive concepts, will ultimately give you positive results.

You have heard the old Biblical adage, "As a man thinketh, so is he."? I used to hear my students when they came in the room on test day mumbling about "I'm going to fail this test!" Fail they did! But when they heeded my advice to relax, open their minds to a positive flow of thoughts, find the trigger words that would spark a memory, and jot a few key things down at the start of the test, then they usually passed even when poorly prepared.

A friend of mine doesn't even believe in saying "I feel like I'm getting sick," because he knows he has planted the seeds of an illness attitude that will flesh out in his becoming ill. I've personally switched to saying, "I feel a little suspicious. Think I'll take some Echinacea, C, and D to ward it off." As a former high school teacher, you can be sure the germs were constantly swirling around me, but getting really sick was not the norm for me.

Reading the *Power of Positive Thinking* by Norman Vincent Peele, reinforced my belief that thoughts are things. Actual things. Objects we cannot see, but can mentally and emotionally feel and see. We've all had the experience of walking into a room, instantly reading the "vibes," or someone saying something you had just thought but had not yet spoken? We read thoughts all of the time; and I do not think it is just reading the body language of those around us. Dr. Peele recommended a little test to prove this concept: next time you are in a group of people, pick out one person and say a positive, affirming prayer for them. They will, most likely, turn toward you, make eye contact, and smile.

So, our wellness on any level boils down to the thought process. How we think about things. What kind of inner dialog are we bathing our minds in, and what are the resulting "vibes"/thoughts that we are sending others? Is this getting too touchy-feely for you? Hang in there! I don't want to sound like a flower child tripping through the tulips, but there is power in our thoughts; and there is power in our words which stem from thoughts.

We have seen the power of our words as they gave friendship, healing, calm, love, and peace. Likewise, we have seen our words inflict pain, hurt, and have even created death in relationships. Our wellness depends upon how we think; and yes, I am saying that we should develop a greater sense of being in harmony with the spheres/universe in order to bring about that wellness.

A perfect area to strengthen your positive connection is with your own body. Before we can control what is going on with our health, we have to establish the proper "conversation tone" about our relationship and responsibility to our body. Keep reading so you can actually DO this in the next section.

Take Away Thoughts:

- Wellness is often depicted as a triangle with each angle equidistant from the next, all parts being equally important. The physical is no good without a brain, and the spiritual/emotional side is thought about, so the mental side must take the lead!

- All health starts with a thought, followed up by what we do with it.

- Thinking gives us tremendous power!

Take Away Actions:

- Harness that power to not only better yourself, but to better your world!

- Practice a positive dialog with yourself.

- Start each day with an affirmation such as, "This is a beautiful day and I will be a part of that beauty in all I say and do!"

This leads us to making a mindset shift.

Mindset Shift

"Your mindset is the foundation of your 'personal house.'
Walls and a roof without a foundation is no more than a tent,
and a tent probably won't withstand heavy rains or high
winds."
—Michal Stawicki, *Master Your Time in 10 Minutes a Day*

Are you just sort of 'along for the ride' with your daily life and resulting health status? Did you know your daily life is even connected to your health? Hopefully, because you are holding this book, you already know there is a real cause-and-effect relationship here. I have seen many people sort of bump along life's highway, doing what everyone else was doing, what the television has us think is "normal," and thinking their less-than-perfect health status was to be expected. Doesn't everyone take pills for high blood pressure, high blood sugar, anti-depressants, bad digestion, gas, bloating, IBS, GERD, ED, and a host of other diseases and conditions? Doesn't everyone eat Pop Tarts, pizza, Hamburger Helper, Pepsi, Coke, McDonald's everything, Fruit Loops? ......Well, "No!"

You are not along for the ride. You are an active participant in your health every moment! You do have power. It's the power of choice!

Understanding and accepting that you hold in your brain vast powers of life and death, let's re-connect with yourself in a more positive, healthful way.

Following Alexandra Jamieson's blog, I have learned about a guided breathing exercise she uses to not only calm down, but to connect with her body. This connection highlights the symbiotic relationship that her beautifully functioning body has with her mind. It also leads her to be mindful and considerate of her body.

Here is my take on Alex's Mindset Shift:

In a quiet room, sit comfortably in a chair. Place one of your hands on your belly and the other hand over your heart. Close your eyes and slowly breathe. Breathe in through your nose and exhale gently through your nose. There's no rush. Breathe in to a count of five and exhale to a count of five. Feel the rise and fall of your hands as they rest on your chest and belly. Keep breathing. Feel the warmth of your hand on your belly. Your hand is giving warmth to your belly and your belly is giving warmth to your hand. Keep breathing. Did you know that the organs in your belly help you in so many different ways beside digestion? They function as a second brain, a second nervous system with lighting fast connections to your brain warning you of dangers. Thank your belly for helping you. Keep breathing as you also thank you belly for protecting you from toxins, germs, and viruses. Feel that warmth beneath your hand spread and grow stronger. Keep breathing as you promise to listen to the needs of your belly because it will never steer you wrong. You want to help it run smoothly to protect your body. You will also protect it. As you keep breathing, feel your heart beat under your other hand. That beautiful heart, always faithful, always beating. Again, feel the warmth under your hand and feel that warmth radiate its glow all over your body, giving it life-sustaining goodness. Thank your heart and promise to take care of it as it is always taking care of you. Keep breathing and acknowledge that you are the sum of your parts and that you are fearfully and wonderfully made! Feel that warmth and be thankful! Keep breathing and then slowly open your eyes.

Try this. In just a couple of minutes you will feel refreshed, connected, and committed in the marvelous and dynamic relationship you have with your whole self.

Take Away Thoughts:

- You can harness great powers within yourself.

- Mindful breathing exercise is easy, quick, and can totally rejuvenate your mind-body-spirit.

- By being in tune with your body, you can recommit your thinking and resultant actions toward the welfare of your whole self. You feel the force of a united team, all aiming toward the same goal of wellness.

- Remember this commitment is...sacred! Only *you* have this commitment, this relationship with your mind-body-spirit. It is to be respected, guarded, and nurtured. We are obliged to better understand how this trinity-of-self works, so we can stay true to our commitment.

Take Away Actions:

- As you quietly reconnect with your inner Self, enjoy the palpable warmth, and even vibration, underneath your hands as they are over your heart and belly. That connection is real as is the promise you make to yourself to 'watch your 6,' so-to-speak. It's a trust thing.

- All day long, ask yourself if what you are doing or eating is doing your body good. If you know it is not, then you need to revisit your commitment. You also need to reexamine your active role in being responsible for yourself.

Knowledge is power, so let's get going!

Stay Connected

Writers spout a lot of good ideas, but do they use those ideas on themselves? Sort of like: "Doctor, heal thyself!" Well yes, I am consciously choosing to have breathing sessions several times a day. This is a new day for me as I write this section of your *Toolkit for Wellness*; and before writing, I reconnected with myself through a very brief breathing session.

I am no different than everyone else—sources of stress abound. After having had a bout of stress-induced cardiomyopathy in 2008, I have had to learn my limits, develop and follow stress reducing techniques, say 'yes' to things that relax me, and say "no' to things that just add to my stress levels. We are all a work-in-progress, to be sure; and through my research, listening, and living, I am more cognizant than ever that I can, I **must** be, **actively** involved in my stress balancing. Inner peace does not plop itself in our laps. We have to actively seek it.

One thing I have to remember is, each day brings new challenges and opportunities. Life is not static and we do not land in a 'good place' and stay there. Everything is in flux and we have to 'read' ourselves, keep our fingers on our 'pulse,' to assess how we are doing. Sometimes, the doing of what we think is keeping us balanced can become a source of stress itself. Writing this book is bringing me great satisfaction, pleasure, and happiness in just knowing that I am getting closer to helping more people than I can teach in just one room. However, all of the components that go into creating a book can sometimes overwhelm and be a source of great pressure. Regularly, I have to re-frame my thinking to avoid having this dear project become a false refuge of stress reduction from my duties as a caregiver.

I am coming to realize this is being called 'mindfulness,' using our minds to engage with ourselves, with our Creator, and with our universe. Just today on the news, I heard the results of yet another study showing that mindful meditation—employing controlled breathing—surpassed the results of the control group for coronary artery disease that used standard medical care! Once you tune into mindfulness, you will pick up all kind of mentions in the news as to its benefits.

This is not a passing fancy. Meditation is centuries old. I just always linked the word 'meditation' with someone sitting cross-legged, hands resting on their knees, fingers in the 'okay' position, and 'omming'...Oh, and snake charmers in the background! I was a bit leery of this because I did not want to join a new religion.

Those misconceptions have held me back, but thanks to some special guidance and suggestions from our daughter and some friends, my meditation time has blossomed...no lotus positions needed! Just recently, I was guided to try a mindfulness meditation audio book; and I have to say, it really helped me step back and approach my day with a new kind of calm. Since I am all about helping through sharing of contacts, you can check this out for yourself at:

https://itunes.apple.com/us/audiobook/finding-true-refuge-meditations/id598842424

I was also aware, the more people prayed, the greater sense of peace they received. Until recently, I confess I was more of just an all-day-say-short-thankful-prayers kind of person. But by combining mindful-breathing and meditation to strip away the multitasking focus that surrounded me, I am better set up to an even richer communion with my Creator than I ever was just closing my eyes to pray.

I always viewed my inability to concentrate in prayer without my mind wandering off as a serious personal character flaw. Now I understand that being plagued by wandering thoughts during prayer was just the result of a flawed technique. Even without meditation, breathe first, reconnect with yourself, experience that releasing from all that tugs for your attention, and then connect with your Creator and with the vibrations of the universe so wondrously made. It then becomes easy to find your prayer focus.

It's all a part of life—being connected—you'll never want to lose that wonderful feeling! Stay connected. In so doing, you will discover the power of choice is even greater than you thought. Maybe my mother's wisdom will help you harness the power of your ability to choose. That's what we will explore next.

Take Away Thoughts:

- Connecting with yourself, calming the voices and distractions around us is not a one-time deal.

- Like any team, your mind-body-spirit team needs to practice each day or the skills learned by your team will grow faint and distant.

- Reconnecting with yourself allows an easier reconnection with your Creator

Take Away Actions:

- Each of us has a special, reflective opportunity every day. Maybe it doesn't happen until a solitary drive to work—in which case, eye closing is out! But whenever your brief moment is, take it! Seize it and hold it near as those moments will transform your day and set you on a positive path. Breathe mindfully and smile!

Now get ready to see just how intentional our thinking is!

A Mother's Wisdom-Mindfulness Applied: It's a Matter of Choice

It wasn't until well into adulthood that I finally absorbed the greatest life lesson my mother ever gave me. "Thank you, Mom!" Of course, at the time she gave me that lesson, I thought she was being overbearing and maybe a bit cruel.

Typical of most teenagers, there were times when I just sort of coasted along while doing my chores. This particular time, I was changing our sheets and making our beds. Simple enough task. I was glad to do it, even. But as I mindlessly drifted through the chore, I put the wrong end of the top sheet at the head of the bed. You know: The wider hem on the top sheet goes at the head of the bed so it will look pretty when turned back over the covers? Well, I did it the wrong way. Mom saw that, mentioned it, and I fixed it. No big deal. Next week, I once again floated through my bed making tasks and repeated my error. Mom was not happy. She said I had done that **on purpose**! Give me a break. I would never have intentionally irritated my mom. I loved her! What an awful blow it was to know she was thinking that about me!

Then she clarified her message. I had, too, done it on purpose because I knew better and **chose not to think**!

What on earth? How do you choose to not think...Why would I do that on purpose? Clearly my mom was weird.

But you know what? I have always chosen to think about what I was doing while making beds from that day on.

"It just happened," will never be an excuse for me.

Clearly, in every single solitary thing I do, I have the choice to engage my brain or not.

It's a heavy responsibility.

I think it's called being an adult.

So, being 'mindful' to me means engaging the brain, understanding, and doing things on purpose—which Mom taught me was ALL of the time—but now, being mindful will make that purpose a positive one. 'Mindfulness' means pausing all of the distractions all about me to reflect on meaning.

To the good or to the bad, every second of life we have a choice, and we are making them.

Recent reading has shown me that we make over 60,000 choices each day. Many of them carry no great consequence, but many of them certainly do. Choosing something that is wrong for our well-being once might not always result in doom, but even a second bad choice starts a pattern. We start habits, good or bad, by repeating a pattern. There is a way to change bad patterns, and it starts with your first tool: Your brain.

Take Away Thoughts:

- Everything we do is on purpose!

- Even little choices can create a pattern and create the start of a habit.

- We all have a choice!

Take Away Actions:

- Waking up and being more aware is awesome! While doing even the repetitive chores, be aware of all the details of what's going on and chose to be responsible for what you are seeing and doing. Isn't that what we wish others were doing?

When others **aren't** choosing to be aware, our stress levels can often rise! Keep reading about some useful and easy-to-use depressurizing tools in your *Toolkit for Wellness*.

AIR, AIR PRESSURE GAUGE, AND RELEASE VALVES

Okay. We all are dealing with a lot of stress. As this conversation continues, I hope to share with you a few tools I have personally used, and have seen others use, to stay grounded even in the midst of stressful storms. If I can give you just one or two ideas to easily incorporate into your daily routine, then I can rest knowing I have helped in some small way. That is what this is all about.

So, let's get going as we revisit a key stress reliever that can stop your stress response in its tracks!

We will also be looking at some relatively easily-fixable specifics that may secretly be contributing to your overall stress without your knowledge. It's all about keeping that number one tool functioning at optimum levels.

We will be learning how finding our "voice" can brighten our outlook and change our lives. No, I don't mean singing in the shower! Although it is a great stress reliever... maybe not to the listeners though.

Now, the oxygen please!

Air!

Air. Breath. Life. They all go together, don't they? Breath IS life. When we mindfully breathe, we are reconnected to the moment, the present, and can revel in the wonder of being alive. Let's deconstruct simple cleansing breaths.

1. It is possible to do this standing, but sitting upright with a straight back in a chair seems to be best. Of course, my yoga friends may find that cross-legged pose even better.

2. Relax your shoulders by dropping them down. We hold so much tension there without even realizing it and lowering our shoulders can relieve a lot of stress right there.

3. Hands comfortably in your lap.

4. Eyes closed.

5. Gently inhale through your nose.

6. Gently exhale through your nose or your slightly parted lips.

7. Feel the movement of air.

8. Think only about the breathing sensation and how it feels. If thoughts invade your space, gently release them for now and return to centering your breath.

9. Now inhale to a count of three, hold the air for a count of three, exhale for a count of three, and pause for a count of three, and then take the next breath.

10. Now inhale to a count of five, hold the air for a count of five, exhale for a count of five, pause for a count of five, and then take the next breath.

After just 5-10 breaths, you can feel the de-stressing relaxation wash over you. You are truly in the moment. You deserve to feel like this. No gym membership needed. A tool you can pull out and use at any time and any place.

Seems as though we are talking about breathing a lot. Indeed! This simple tool will not only transform your stress response right now, but will invigorate your whole body with improved oxygenation and toxin removal. I have read that mindful breathing will actually put you into the perfect metabolic state. Getting there is a breath away!

Take Away Thoughts:

- With daily application, this mindful breathing can actually be used to stop your stress response in its tracks. Remove yourself from a situation, get by yourself for a moment, and mindfully breathe. Don't use that time to rehash things or think of how you are going to react or act. Just breathe. It takes some practice, but doing this at least once a day will give you a valuable tool in times of great stress.

Take Away Actions:

- Give yourself a happy 'ah' moment by starting the day with this simple technique to help 'clean the slate' for a new beginning.

- Just sitting down to your desk at work to dive into today's activities? There is time for you to take five mindful breaths! Do it now—it will transform how you feel about your day ahead.

Let's see now what everyone's Pressure Gauge is reading. Are we pegging those meters? Is there any help? Of course, keep reading!

Pressure Gauge

How's your pressure gauge reading? Pegged? How can you tell? Oh, let's see:

- Tired

- Poor sleep

- Sleeping all of the time

- Poor concentration

- Eating extra carbohydrates—sweets, breads, cakes, canned drinks

- High blood pressure

- Poor digestion

- Unusual weight loss or gain

- Testy relations with those around you

- Feelings of helplessness and hopelessness

- Inability to concentrate

- No time for yourself

How are we doing? We've all been there. Circumstances do happen. Jobs are lost, bills are due, cars break down, and flood waters do rise. Bad things happen to good people. There are no magic wands and life isn't simple, I know; but maybe we can put a few tools into your hand that will help you cope.

Stress. Pressure. That which vexes us. There is even the pressure of *good* things that can push our limits.

Where does your stress come from? Is it primarily from within? ...from without? ...or a combination of both? Does it matter?

You bet! But we can't deal with our stressors until we come to an understanding of what they actually are.

Oh, the problem is that everyone needs something from me. There are so many deadlines, I can't keep up! Oh, why is that? Maybe after pausing to reconnect with yourself and examine your stress, you can find ways to look at things differently and see there **are** ways to free yourself. Let's take a look at Release Valves.

Finding YOUR voice in a Release Valve and a Five Step Plan

We all have an inner dialog going on, but are there other voices, too? Voices from the past? Imagined voices of the future? If there's one thing I am learning from mindful breathing sessions, it's those sessions bring me firmly into the present, the now.

Now is the only thing we have to live, the only thing we can impact. Can't put a dent in the past. Can't totally control tomorrow. But I can live right now; and in so doing, I might be able to color the future just a bit, but I can't *absolutely* control the future. Certainly, lessons learned from the past should be incorporated into our "now" to prevent making repeated mistakes and assist in planning; but plans without the actions of "now" are useless.

We are left with today; but our quiet time thoughts today are often crowded out by a "voice committee"—you know; those 'voices' from the past? Who or what is monopolizing the conversation in your head?

Wringing your emotional hands over the past is fixing absolutely nothing but is certainly robbing you of your Now.

Time is our only true commodity, the only thing we have to give: Our time, our *now*. Acting on the truth that none of us is guaranteed a tomorrow, should push us to not fritter away our only 'now' by dawdling over something which we have no power to change.

Letting go is a nice idea, but it's easier said than done! Follow Karl Moore's suggestion in his delightful book, *The 18 Rules of Happiness*, and try this:

Take several deep cleansing breaths and ask yourself if you could just let go of that negative thought or emotion just for today. Just for right now. A 'yes' or a 'no' is all you need. If you are somehow not ready to let go, fine. Revisit the question tomorrow. There is no judgment of your choice. If the answer is 'yes,' then as you take in the next breath and exhale, also release that negative feeling. Feel the release. The letting go will leave you feeling lighter and freer.

Free to find your own voice, one that fits you right now—not yesterday, not tomorrow. Now.

This is a process of gradually uncluttering your mind from the "voice committee." Those other voices are not the ones living your life—you are. Claim it! We give power to those voices when we hash and re-hash negative experiences. Of course, it is possible to give power to even those positive experiences from the past by literally living in the past all of the time.

Listen to your own actual conversations with others. Are they centered solely on past experiences and people who are long gone? What are you doing with your life right now? What are you working on right now? What are you reading? What are you doing? You. Now. Not with your long gone family and friends, but with you and those who live right now.

A widow friend of mine shared, as she worked through her grief in dealing with the loss of her husband, she was admittedly living in the past quite a bit. Her sister rather rudely and hurtfully exclaimed she needed to move on, her husband was dead! While not advocating such an abrupt confrontation, she eventually took the message to heart. Slowly, she stopped dwelling on the past, and started a totally refreshing rediscovery of her own self. What did **she** want to do? Where did **she** want to go? How did **she** want to grow? Having dropped voices from the past, she discovered her own voice! In reflection, it was the first time in her whole life she was finally listening to **her** inner voice. She couldn't smile enough!

The Five Step Plan

So many of us get caught up in wishful planning. I call them "wishful plans" because they are never followed by actions.

Inaction can seriously contribute to the stress of perceived failure. Little is out of our reach as long as we persevere in taking those tiny daily steps that will lead us to our goals. Do you have a dream? Then let me share five steps I have taken that helped me realize mine. These steps are easy to follow and have helped me realize and find my voice. My dream? You are holding it!

1. Acknowledge your dream. Everyone has one or more. Far too many never take it to the next step. There are countless stories about people who have overcome all sorts of astounding odds to make their dreams a reality. Michal Stawicki and Jeannie Ingraham's book, *99 Perseverance Success Stories*, is an inspiring collection of short stories about everyday people who mastered taking daily steps to get to their goals. No handicap or poor circumstance could stop their perseverance from succeeding.

2. Regularly tap into sources of inspiration. It does take a village to do anything. Use the vast amount of positive energy around you and stay inspired. My resources are many.

   Church is my first. In worship, I am reminded we are all gifted by God with talents that He wants us to use. If our talents help people, we are a success.

I began teaching my first *Designed for Health* class after hearing a familiar sermon message that God has a plan for us and we have to step out in faith. Dr. Dan Day explained to our congregation that God will equip us to carry out the message He wants us to give to help others. Every week, people were coming to me with health and wellness questions. Was I going to ignore my talents and not help others on a grander scale?

Another source is James Clear, who inspired me to start my own blog. His sends out a weekly message about habit formation and perseverance. His tips in November of 2014 about starting a blog inspired me to step out of my comfort level and *do it*! I continue to thank him.

Search for books that will inspire you and move you to self-growth. Author Michal Stawicki, whom I have already mentioned, has been a real spring board for me to believe in my dream, take tiny consistent steps, and persevere. His books, *Art of Perseverance,* and, *Trickle Down Mindset,* have given me tremendous boosts in my path to self-improvement and fulfillment.

Claire Cook's book, *Never Too Late: Your Roadmap to Reinvention,* inspired me as a writer. She tells the story of how she wrote her first novel sitting in a cold car before dawn while waiting on her daughter at ice skating practice. That book not only became a best seller, but a first-rate award winning movie!

3. Break down your project into smaller pieces. This dream of yours may become a ten year project, but do not get lost squinting your eyes at the goal so far away.

Look instead on today's goal. Check off today's goal and then take the next step tomorrow. Daily movement. Daily action. Daily steps. Not ruminating that the goal is so far away it is impossible. Break it down.

4. Learn as much as possible about how to achieve steps to your dream. With the Internet, the world is at our fingertips. Take advantage of this by looking into what you want to do. I continue to learn about nutrition and wellness on a daily basis, but writing a book? I knew how to write, but how to get my ideas from here to there? I began to follow various websites, subscribing to them, learning all I could for free. Then, amongst the many how-to-write-and-publish sites came one that stood out above the others. Chandler Bolt put on a massive webinar summit for writers. It included many people I had been following and respected. I decided to join his Self-Publishing School to seal the deal, learn the last part, and complete my journey as a first time author. If you want to write, visit this link to his free video about writing:
https://xe172.isrefer.com/go/firstbook/DJEdwards

5. Take tiny steps every day. I could stop right there. Without moving everyday toward your goal, you are going nowhere. Inaction is the same as taking the first step backwards. Inaction can reverse the tide of having done all of your good work. One miss may be okay, but two? Two misses is a pattern.

So, there is my Five-Step Plan for success! Sounds like another book....

Take Away Thoughts:

• Ponder the words from a sage of long ago, Marcus Aurelius, in his writings called "Meditations":

"Casting aside other things, hold to the precious few; and besides, bear in mind that every man lives only the present, which is an invisible point, and that all the rest of his life is either past or is uncertain."

- The need to concentrate on the "now" is as relevant as it was around 188 AD! We live in that thin line called "now." Claim it and do not give it away!

Take Away Actions:

- Listen to yourself talk. Are you talking about the past more than you are talking about the present? Have you left all of your accomplishments in the past? In this ever-changing world, there's always something new to learn, to see, to hear, or to do. Look around for **today's** activities.

- Find **your** voice in fulfilling **your** dream. It is never too late to start!

- Follow the Five-Step Plan to realize your dream by:

  1. Acknowledging it,

  2. Tapping into inspiration,

  3. Breaking down your goal to small doable steps,

  4. Learning as much as possible, and

  5. Taking tiny steps every day

But wait! There's more! Continue reading to find *more* ways to calm the inner merry-go-round so you can focus your efforts for action.

More Stress Relief Valves

Mindful breathing—which is my go-to quick remedy for immediate stress reduction—is just one of many methods to lower stress. There are countless other ways people find that stress release button.

You have felt the immediate release that can come from just stepping out of doors. The limitless boundaries of space somehow release those problems and concerns that had been crushing us while inside the four walls. Being in nature has to be the most natural stress reliever in the world. Whenever possible, we all should strive to be outdoors, breathing in the fresh air, gazing at the sky and clouds, opening up to the sounds of nature, and the buzz of life around us.

A simple trip to the mail box can take several minutes while I stroll in the sunlight around the house. What a relaxing time it is! I literally just did this as a break from writing today. Grab a hold of some pure bliss while merely getting the mail.

Certainly, we have all developed our own ways to lighten any moment or pause our busy days: Exercise (there's a whole chapter on that), music, reading, a quiet bath, knitting, painting, golfing (although that can also be a serious point of stress, too), and whatever hobby or activity that brings you pleasure or calmness.

Even relaxing on the back porch is great, but sometimes I see weeds to pull or flowers that need watering. Help! What to do? If you are looking for a tool to turn down the inner stress levels, I have another one. I do this with my eyes wide open and with my mind tuned into something totally different. This activity is, at once, fully engaging my senses but not contributing to added stress. It is akin to comfort food, but without the calories, sugar, fat, guilt, or health consequences.

It creates deep down comfort that hails from our childhood. Remember sitting down with a brand new box of crayons and a new coloring book? I will never forget moving up to that 64-color pack of Crayola wonderfulness! Through the years, I have often thought that some days would have been made perfect by coloring to relieve those stressful moments in life. But I wanted adult pictures and maybe quality colored pencils! Well, why not?

Recently, Parade magazine featured an article on a growing trend for adult coloring books. Vaguely aware of this smart return to adult coloring needs, I read with relish about resources now available to answer that inner desire to focus, not on learning the latest technology or social media app, but to just apply color to the page.

They even gave a free resource at parade.com/coloring where you can download and print a few sample pictures and designs to get started. After a trip to the craft store, I returned home with new set of 24-count colored pencils. I started to give life to a pretty picture of paper lanterns, streamers, and dangling beads.

Right now, my coloring station is easily accessible on an open space of the kitchen counter. It has become a favorite spot to start my day—after doing planks—and a new way to finish my evening winding down process before bed. It's amazing what just five minutes of coloring can do for one's mind and spirit.

There is no multi-tasking with applying color to paper. There is no half-hearted or distracted effort here. Coloring gently requires our full attention. The only thing I am thinking about is applying the chosen color to the paper in a way that pleases me. It is completely engaging, yet not stressful in nature. It's like meditating with your eyes wide open.

There are repetitive patterns available such as paisley prints or mandalas, and there are pictures as well, such as "The Secret Garden." The Parade link will give you a variety to choose from so you can experiment with the coloring experience before actually buying a full book.

Crayons, markers, pastels, or colored pencils—it does not have to be complicated. Certain markers may bleed and crayons quickly get rounded points—that's why I went with colored pencils.

Another calming effect with this coloring activity is, it enables me to organize and put order to the page. I have seen and heard of people who rely on jig-saw puzzles to help them to have a sense of putting their lives back in order during or after stressful or traumatizing events. With coloring, I think the therapeutic power is magnified because there is also a creative process going on. Rather than piecing together a picture someone else created, you are giving color, life, order, and beauty to something to which you actively contributed.

If you can give life, color, and beauty to a printed design, then maybe you can do the same in a certain area of your life! In any case, you will leave from the coloring experience much more relaxed and with a stronger inner calm to either face the day or to ease into a restful sleep.

Take Away Thoughts:

- So, there you have it. The bottom line is actually using any of these stress reduction activities. It's our choice to make. Ultimately, we run our lives and we need to claim the calm we were designed to have.

- Practicing the use of these calming tools on a day-to-day basis will make it easier to turn to them in times of crisis.

Take Away Actions:

- Sometimes we have to say out loud to ourselves, "Stop!" before we spin out of control. You are not alone. I did that this week. Out loud. "Stop!" followed by my affirmations of, "Fear not," and, "Peace I give to you," and when I got back home...I colored. Smile!

Sometimes our Toolkits get jumbled up over time. Check out how jumbled efforts and environments can affect our spirits. Next up: some tips on how to put things in order internally and externally.

Keeping the Toolkit Organized

De-cluttering can occur on many planes. Think of your tool kit as having been left open in the shop over the years, its neatness and cleanliness being degraded with wood shavings, dust, dirt, oil, and the scrambling of tools as they were carelessly tossed back in. Talk about clutter!

Getting rid of those extra voices and discovering your own voice is just the beginning to overall wellness. How are those flat surfaces doing around your house or at work? Can you even find them? I have a tendency to fill up flat surfaces, too; but the pure enjoyment I get from clean surfaces is so great, keeping the majority of my counters and tables cleaned off is relatively easy.

My retirement from public education coincided with my husband's declining health and pushed me to take over the household bills, paperwork, and filing. Oh, my husband filed alright, bless his heart; but his files were stacks and stacks of papers and envelopes which encroached my kitchen counters! Jumanji! Ack! Once I set up a small box of files with the current year's receipts and pared down what was saved for the long term (with a new definition of long-term), I felt as though the very air was cleaner, clearer, and lighter.

Scientific studies have shown that people are more productive in cleaner, less cluttered environments. Even if you are a messy type person, carve out an area at your work desk and de-clutter what is in your line of sight. You will immediately notice how much easier it is to start work and stay focused. Visual distraction from clutter clogs the mind.

A further epiphany occurred with a recent installation of new wall-to-wall carpeting throughout the house (even closets). While never one to actively acquire collections of things, there were many mementos amassed from living in the same house for nearly 35 years, raising two children, returning to college for nursing, teaching for 17 years, collecting partial household goods from both sides of our family, and retiring from teaching and from a home-based video production business. All of this stuff had to go somewhere. Can you imagine cleaning out every nook and cranny of your house and not moving? Try it!

I am enjoying the openness and the free, flat surfaces so much that 90% of the nonessential stuff I moved out will never return. Stuff can eat you alive. It creeps in around you, slowly but surely getting a choke hold around your neck and holding your very 'essence' hostage. Besides, dusting is a cinch without having to move and dust objects just to get to the surface they are on.

Oh, and the hanging portraits, pictures and memorabilia of our now adult children had never changed. Parents: Is your home a shrine to the kids when they were little? While those moments in time are treasures to any parent, hasn't your role in this world moved on since you went to the piano recitals and little league games? Does your home reflect your 'now' voice? Our children totally approved our new look, devoid of their elementary school accomplishments. Liberate those picture frames, file or give away the pictures, and refresh them with "today," and ....maybe not have as many sitting around needing dusting.

Are there relationships or obligations that are cluttering your life? If you are giving more than you are getting from those relationships, it is time for de-cluttering that area of your life, too. Remember, our time, our 'now,' is the only thing we have to give. If those obligations are no longer reflecting who you are or what you want to be about, then letting them go will free you up to choose those things and people that more truly reflect who you are now.

As we start talking about de-cluttering our eating habits, we will be addressing kitchen cupboards, continuing to surround ourselves with foods that generate 'dis-ease' forces us to dip into our limited resources of will power. We are going to be all about habit development, not willpower development; so, ridding the cupboards of temptations will be high on our lists. More on that later.

Take Away Thoughts:

- While some stress cannot be stopped, we can control our reactions to it.

- De-cluttering our minds helps us find our 'voice.'

- De-cluttering relationships and obligations is probably something we all need to do occasionally as we change through time.

- De-cluttering our physical environment can help our minds and spirits, too.

Take Away Actions:

- Take a moment for calm breathing. Listen to any negative thoughts that may slip in. Ask yourself if you would be willing, just for today, to release that negative thought? If the answer is 'yes," then as you breathe out, consciously and physically release that thought. Enjoy that release!

- Get back to the present time, the now, to find your 'now' voice.

- Pick a small area of your home to de-clutter today. Hard to choose where to begin? Start around where you are seated.

- Challenge: Partner with a friend and commit to throwing or giving away things for thirty days. One item on day one. Two items on day two until, on day thirty, you give or throw away thirty items. This could be a great spring or fall cleaning challenge that a group of friends or family members could do with a celebratory party at the conclusion!

Next, we will be looking at the tool of an "Owner's Manual." You know, the last thing we read knowing it should have been the first thing? Maybe we are just too stubborn to read the directions? That's okay. I've got you covered!

OWNER'S MANUAL

We are not born with an owner's manual, are we? Our parents wish we were. It's no small task raising a child, being responsible for his/her total care 24-7. It's no easy task taking charge of our own care either; but much can be gained by a basic understanding of some anatomy and physiology.

My Health Occupations students were full of questions about how their bodies worked. In fact, when you gather people of any age, they are brimming with questions about physiological processes and health. Teaching anatomy was so fun, and it remains a favorite topic of personal study. The part of this very large field I want to share with you here is the digestive system because how we take care of that system affects the whole body.

First, let me introduce the concept of wavy versus straight lines. The best way to go from point A to point B is a straight or smooth line if the function is, say, covering an organ or the body. Our skin is smooth. Our heart, lungs, and intestines are covered with smooth tissue to protect and enhance their motile functioning.

But if surface area is needed, say, in our brain, a straight or smooth line of brain matter would not give us enough cerebral cortex or gray matter to have much tissue with which to think. Hence the wavy, folded surface of our brain which allows for increased surface area! Little known fact that could help you in a quiz show: If we could 'iron out" the surface area of our brain, we would end up with the area of a pillow case. Now that's brain power!

Let's consider the digestive system.

Mouth: Smooth inside with teeth and tongue for chewing, tasting and swallowing functions. Home to salivary glands that start the moistening process so we do not swallow dry toast. Saliva also starts the early breaking down of carbohydrates.

Throat and esophagus: Smooth inside for the transport of mushy, swallowed food.

Stomach: Smooth but folded to allow for expansion and churning actions to break down food. Contractions of stomach muscles combine the moist swallowed food with stomach acids that also aid in the breakdown process, killing moderate amounts of bacteria and other toxins.

Small intestine: Not smooth because *much* surface area is needed for exposing the soup-like foodstuffs to the intestinal wall. It is here that most of the absorption of nutrients occurs. I have heard Dr. Tom O'Bryan describe the small intestine as a shag carpet surface. The shag carpet projections are called villi and the fuzzy parts of each villi are called microvilli. It is this area we will talk about the most, the health and well-being of those little villi and microvilli is ground zero for most of our health issues!

Liver, pancreas, and gall bladder: Important accessory organs to the digestive system that add their goodies for the digestive process at the beginning of the small intestine.

The liver with its over two hundred functions is a vital organ we cannot live without. It makes the bile, which is stored and delivered by the gall bladder. The liver serves as the collection and processing center of all of the nutrients taken into the body from the small intestine, before releasing them to the general circulation. The liver also performs a host of functions involved with metabolism, such as removing alcohol from the blood, and storing energy in the form of glycogen for quick release to the body when needed.

Pancreatic juices enhance the digestive process by producing enzymes that help digest protein, and makes buffers to neutralize stomach acids. The pancreas also supplies the hormone insulin, which is needed to balance out blood sugar spikes when carbohydrates are eaten by delivering glucose to the cells.

The gall bladder squirts out the bile made in the liver, which helps with the effective breakdown and absorption of fats.

Large intestine a.k.a. colon: Smooth surface and home to more micro-organisms than there are cells in our bodies! It's a regular shoot out at the OK Corral in there. Hopefully, the good guys are winning! Our immune response and the homeostasis/balancing of body functions is dependent upon this microbiome.

Another big function of the large intestines is to extract the water in the 'soup' leftover from the digestive process. People who have had their entire colon removed have serious concerns with staying hydrated. That's how important the large intestine is in terms of water balance!

Rectum: Smooth but folded for expansion. Serves as a 'holding tank' for the final leftovers from digestion.

Anal canal and anus: The exit point for the leftovers a.k.a. feces, #2, and poop. There is much to be learned about the shape and texture of this, too, but later.

Hormones that Control Appetite, Satiety, and How We Burn Fats

So, you have been introduced to the digestive system. Time to say 'hello' to the hormones that control our eating habits and how we burn fat.

Meet ghrelin. It's the hormone that says, "I'm hungry!" Ghrelin is produced in the stomach lining, pancreas, and in the brain. Stress and sleep deprivation cause *more* ghrelin to be released, thus causing increased hunger and a desire for carbohydrates during those times.

While there is just one hunger hormone—ghrelin—there are three signals to let us know we are full! Leptin is the first. Produced in white fat tissue and in the stomach lining, leptin not only says, "I'm full!" but also increases our metabolic rate *and* fat burning for energy needs! Adiponectin is another, "I'm full," signaler from fat tissue; and interestingly enough, thin people produce more.

Finally, there is a Peptide called YY, produced in the small intestine that increases the body's sensitivity to the, "I'm full," signals from leptin. The foods that contain protein and fat cause a lot of this peptide to be released. Carbohydrates cause little to be released. Thus, there is more satiety in protein and (good) fat consumption than in carbohydrate consumption.

Understanding the interplay of these hunger and satiety factors should cause us to rethink snack and meal choices. Carbohydrates will not satisfy which causes overeating. Protein and good fat choices, say, a handful of nuts or some avocado, will do the job.

Gee, I bet you have 10 questions already! See how much fun science is? This is by no means a complete representation of the digestive system, but this rudimentary foundation will do you well in understanding how to better nourish your body.

The goal, of course, will be to keep this system running as it was designed to do, giving us the health it was designed to give. We were designed for health.

Take Away Thoughts:

- The digestive system is very important, not only in terms of extracting nutritive substances from what we eat, but also in our body-wide balancing of extremes: Good/bad, hydrated/dehydrated, hormones signaling hunger/fullness, low/high blood sugar, and health/disease just to name a few.

- Clearly, a huge focus for our wellness energies needs to be spent on finding and maintaining our digestive health.

Next, we will get down to the nitty-gritty of—well, the "ins and outs". It's super important; but not often discussed. Learn why a conversation about the "ins and outs" is so vital for wellness.

The Ins and Outs

A discussion about the anatomy and physiology of the digestive system—our second brain, the seat of our immune response, and absorber of all nutrition—would be incomplete without addressing the ins and outs. You know, what goes in must come out? In one end and out the other? Food and fluids in. Urine and feces out... or pee and poo, if you will.

Not a dinner table topic of discussion perhaps, unless you are medically employed; but a topic that is of great interest and importance to all of us!

My high school students certainly had a lot of questions that reflected much misunderstanding and lack of knowledge. Girls, especially, were astonished to learn that their twice or three times a day pattern of urination was not normal! Did you know your daughters and granddaughters were doing this? They resort to this Spartan habit because they do not want to use the nasty restrooms at school; a topic to be discussed with your daughters and shared with the principal perhaps.

Talk about a recipe for urinary tract infections today, and a host of other complications now and later in life. I shudder to think of their chronically dehydrated state and/or enormously stretched bladders.

The best measure of how hydrated we are, is not in a count of how many glasses of water or whatever else we drink. The best measure is in the color of the urine. Urine should be clear and lightly colored yellow or amber (like beer). The color will change throughout the day, with it being more intense and concentrated in color first thing in the morning after not drinking all night.

As fluids are introduced throughout the day, the color should quickly change to a lighter, clear yellow. If your urine is practically invisible in the water, perhaps you are too hydrated. It is possible to drink too much water, which will result in a washing away of vital components we need to retain.

If your urine is any color other than some shade of yellow/amber, you need to immediately report this to your doctor for evaluation. No redness; and not the color of brewed tea.

Remember clarity. Urine should always be clear. Cloudy urine needs to be reported to the doctor and tested as well.

Okay. Another area of confusion or misunderstanding involves feces. Poo. Number 2.

Citing my students again, there were many students who thought having a bowel movement once a week was normal. Looking at their chronic dehydration and heavy reliance on the Standard American Fast Food/Junk Food Diet, I could understand this.

We wonder why colon cancer is on the rise.

What's the difference between constipation and the other extreme, diarrhea? A few factors are in play here, namely: 1) water/hydration, 2) fiber, and 3) exercise. This is all powered by the internal movements of our digestive system call peristalsis.

On a day-to-day basis, we may not appreciate the sequential squeezing of our digestive system which, as you learned, is just a long tube with shape changes along the way. Using the analogy of a thirty-foot length of pliable tubing, how are we going to get a 'glump' of mushy foodstuffs along the tube? By sequentially squeezing muscles in the tube from near o far.

Perhaps you have had an intestinal virus when you could feel those squeezes? You try out a bite or two of solid food, maybe dry toast, hoping it will stay down and inside of you. But no! That severe cramping you felt on the way to the rest room was very strong and rapid peristalsis. What you ate was unable to stay in you long enough for the colon to reabsorb the moisture. Diarrhea again!

The flip side of this coin is constipation. As peristalsis is slowed down, the end products stay in the dehydrating colon too long. Passage of such bowel movements can be traumatic.

We seek a happy medium. The best scale to measure and describe this is using the Bristol Stool Form scale a.k.a. the BSF. The BSF originated in the Bristol Royal Infirmary in Bristol, England. The scale describes stools/bowel movements as having seven types:

Type 1: Separate hard lumps, hard to pass

Type 2: Sausage-shaped but lumpy

Type 3: Sausage-like but with cracks on the surface

Type 4: Like a sausage or snake, smooth and soft

Type 5: Soft blobs with clear-cut edges, easy to pass

Type 6: Fluffy pieces with ragged edges, a mushy stool

Type 7: Watery, no solid pieces. Entirely liquid

Type 4 or 5 is what most consider ideal. Certainly, a person with hemorrhoids may have to be content with Type 6, but clean up can be problematic.

If a person is having once a week bowel movements, it's highly unlikely to be a Type 4 or 5. There are direct correlations linking chronic constipation as seen in Type 1 and 2, and colon cancer! Maintaining a Type 4 or 5 can be a daily or twice daily event.

Going back to the three things that contribute to regularity:

1. Water/hydration

2. Fiber

3. Exercise

We have to appreciate how each of these three helps the other. Water keeps things running; fiber keeps things physically manageable, and exercise helps with peristalsis—that forward movement.

With the anti-inflammatory diet that will be outlined later, you will have all of the fibrous ingredients you will need through the vegetable, nut, seed, and fruit components. For an added boost, see the chia seed section in the Starter Recipe chapter.

As described in the Starter Exercises chapter, walking is an exercise available to most all of us. I consider walking a major gut massage, helping with peristalsis, and contributing to regularity.

Take Away Thoughts:

- Conversations about elimination need to be undertaken. Monitor not just yourself, but your family members. Discuss with your medical care provider what your concerns are and **always** report *any* appearance of blood in either urine or stool.

Take Away Actions:

- Monitor the color and clarity of your urine throughout the day. Hydrate appropriately to lighten the color to a pale yellow/amber.

- Strive for Type 4 or 5 by getting enough water, fiber, and exercise.

- Remember that glass of water first thing each morning to get "things" going!

Now that we have covered our digestive anatomy and some related hormone and elimination concerns, let's turn to how the food we eat breaks down. Learning and understanding about the big and small components of food will give you additional insight into what direction your diet needs to go to be "user friendly."

Why are you eating? To just fill up? Or to provide nutrition? Just today in Walmart, I overheard an employee state that she was "Just going to grab a bag of chips and a soda and 'be done' with her lunch." I wanted to weep and put this book into her hands, but it's not quite finished yet! We could put water into our automobile gas tank to just 'fill it up,' but the engine is not going to run. Remember, we are feeding our engines.

BIG WRENCHES AND SMALL WRENCHES

Big Wrenches—Macro-nutrients

We also have to understand how our food is built; or just what are we getting out of our food? Whether eating a green salad, a taco, or a jelly donut, the food we eat has to be broken down to its smallest elements for it to do us any good...or harm...

What we eat is whole and is immediately started on its journey to be broken down at every stop along the way by our digestive system. What we get are the "big wrenches": the macro-nutrients, and the very "small wrenches": micro-nutrients. Protein, fat, and carbohydrates are the "big three wrenches."

Protein

Protein provides building materials for our muscles and our entire body. Growth and tissue repair go on every day in our bodies; and the protein we eat supports this as well as proper immune function, making hormones and enzymes, and providing energy. Essential amino-acids are the building blocks of protein inside our bodies. We need those essential amino acids from our diets to live. Our bodies cannot construct them from other sources. Eating meat, fish, and fowl provides the necessary supply of protein for the human body.

Animal sources of protein contain all of the essential amino acids that we need. Animal sources are all of the meats, plus poultry, fish and eggs. Remember the old commercial about the "incredible, edible egg"? Eggs are the perfect meal in that they have all of the essential amino acids in one little orb! Conventional wisdom has taken a roller coaster ride with that poor egg. There was a time when we were told to hold down egg consumption to just a couple eggs a week. Lately, scientists' reports have released eggs from such artificial restriction.

Plant sources of protein from various vegetables, nuts, and seeds can add to the overall protein count, but do not confer all of the essential amino acids.

Writers and researchers such as Mark Sisson and Robb Wolf, more than amply explain how a diet more closely resembling the balance of macro-nutrients consumed by our primal ancestors, which included a goodly amount of protein, will not result in clogged arteries. The Standard American Diet (SAD) which relies on great quantities of starchy carbohydrates, whole grains, highly-processed vegetable oils, sugar, and high fructose corn syrup *does* lead to clogged arteries.

But eating just any kind of meat will not contribute to our wellness if we do not also look at its source. Feed-lot raised animals are not only given antibiotics and hormones, which translate and contribute to human antibiotic resistance and hormone issues, but they are fed a diet that is primarily corn— to fatten them up. These animals were not meant

to be crammed in shoulder-to-shoulder eating grains. Since when do cows eat grains? They were meant to eat grasses on the range! Just like we are what we eat, they are what they eat, too. They have to be full of stress due to their feed-lot existence, causing total pollution of their bodies (muscles) with stress hormones.

Free range, grass fed, and grass-finished meats are more expensive it's true, but try getting together with another family or two to buy meats in bulk whenever possible. I will share resources for this at the end of the book. In the meantime, check for specials at your local farmer's market.

If you cannot eat the best sourced meats right now, you will still greatly benefit from the better balance of foods outlined in this book. There is no reason to delay making these gradual changes to your diet and lifestyle. The positive outcomes will naturally spur you on to better choices over time...because you will be hooked on feeling great.

Fats

There are essential fatty acids we must get from our diets in order to live. The idea of a fat-free diet is insane! Not only will you miss out on the essential fatty acids, but there are vitamins—the fat soluble Vitamins A, D, E, and K—that need to be consumed with fat in order to be absorbed by the body.

Fat provides for energy and structural integrity. If you are a devotee of the government's food guidelines, the idea of fat actually being needed in the diet represents a big shift in thinking. Hang in there to understand the reasons for 'good' fats being in a healthy diet.

Those thoughts about fat and fat guidelines arose from a study that was totally misrepresented to enhance a desired outcome and dates back to 1953. If you desire a detailed expose on how food guidelines were mishandled and outright manipulated by the politicos and agricultural money, I refer you to, *Death by Food Pyramid,* by Denise Minger.

Truth is, we do need fat in our diets. Every cell of our body has fat molecules in its outer membrane to help hold itself together. Scientific voices that had given proof over and over that saturated fat was *not* the causative factor for coronary heart disease were drowned out by those who preferred to hear something more to their liking. Mention saturated fat today, and everyone naturally thinks it equals certain death.

What *does* equal certain death are the "Franken-fats" which have been developed since modern man got in the mix of playing around with fats at the start of the 1900s. Prior to that, people consumed butter, lard, and animal fat found in meats, fish, poultry, and sea food. Afterwards, the resulting highly processed vegetable oils have been the hallmark of modernism and, oh may I say...the start of a highly *inflammatory* diet that helped kick off *modern* diseases including heart disease.

What this highly processed oil has done is change the balance of Omega-3 and Omega-6 fatty acid ratios from the historical balance of 1:1, to the modern-day balance of 1:10, to even 1:30. We are awash in Omega-6 fatty acids. Overall, Omega-3 fatty acids work to calm inflammation and Omega-6 fatty acids are pro-inflammatory.

We need to shift our fat focus from highly processed fat found in in fast food, packaged foods, and vegetable cooking oils, to fats that are a benefit to us in their purity and their natural fatty acid-balance profile.

The good fats are found in Extra Virgin Olive Oil (the real stuff sold in dark bottles), avocado oil, and coconut oil. Avocado and coconut oil have a higher smoke point than olive oil, and so are better suited for high-heat, stir-fry style cooking. Save using olive oil regularly for salads and sautéing. The light taste of avocado oil also makes it a natural to use by itself for a tossed salad.

Other good oils are found in nuts and seeds. A small handful of nuts can be a powerhouse of a snack. Just remember to start with raw nuts and activate them as instructed in the recipe section to maximize their benefits and make them more digestible. If you see seeds advertised as "sprouted," that means they have already been activated by the soaking and dehydrating process.

Carbohydrates

Carbohydrates provide for energy but there are NO essential carbohydrates that we need from our diets. In fact, our body, itself, can create the carbohydrates that we need for body processes and fuel.

Should we go carb-free? Absolutely not! But there are carbs; and then there are carbs.

Whether you are eating a cupcake, a baked potato, a serving of dark leafy greens, an apple, or you are guzzling sweet iced tea, whatever carbohydrate you put in your body, digestion breaks those carbohydrates down to their simplest form: glucose. Carbohydrates, by definition, all call for a release of insulin which will transport the molecules of glucose out of the blood stream and into the body cells for energy.

The brain and blood cells prefer glucose as their energy form of choice. Any glucose that our cells do not need for immediate use is stored as glycogen in the liver and muscles for future reference. If there is excess glucose beyond storage capability, then it is stored as fat.

Fat burning will *not* occur *first* when our activity levels demand more "gas." No, the energy from the muscles and the liver's glycogen stores will be used first. This is why insulin is called the hormone of fat storage. Eating protein and even good fats will not make your fat cells fatter; eating carbohydrates will.

Glucose is the sugar molecule the body can use for energy. Some carbs take a longer time to break down into glucose. They are said to be complex carbohydrates or carbohydrates with a low glycemic index. In other words, blood sugar levels will not take a big "hit" right away because of the slower conversion rate of carbs to sugar (glucose). The body will run with a steady flow of energy.

These desirable complex carbohydrates are found in the bounty of vegetables, especially dark green leafy greens (salad greens, kale, chard, collards, and spinach to name a few), broccoli, Brussels sprouts, cabbage, and root vegetables such as carrots, radishes, parsnips, turnips, beets, as well as okra, bell peppers, summer and winter squash, and sweet potatoes in moderation. Fruits that are low on the glycemic index include all of the berries with strawberries bringing the highest levels of sugar.

There are other carbohydrates we eat which result in a rapid breakdown into glucose. These carbohydrates cause a big "hit" of blood sugar, which will demand more insulin to be released right away to help transport the glucose load into the body. Such simple carbohydrate-containing foods are said to have a high-glycemic index.

Simple carbohydrates come from the more starchy vegetables—particularly white potatoes, and sweeter fruits such as pineapple, dates, grapes and raisins, from anything made with grain-based flour such as bread, cake, cookies, pasta, and anything made with sugar: cakes, cookies, colas, sweet teas.

Eliminating sugar from the diet can be a bit tricky if you are used to eating any kind of packaged, prepared food. With over forty names for sugar, including high-fructose corn syrup, label reading is a must! Better yet, buy whole foods. There are no labels on apples or carrots.

The trouble with this high-glycemic index scenario is that these carbohydrates will cause great shifts in blood sugar levels from very high to very low; and the body, over time, is more likely to become resistant to the effects of insulin. This is called insulin resistance.

Furthermore, after eating a meal with a great deal of simple carbohydrates, the body feels sluggish, tired, pulled down, and that body will be hungry again sooner because of the resulting blood sugar crash...*if* the insulin is still doing its job to lower blood sugar.

Take Away Thoughts:

- Remember, we were *designed for health*. If human kind was as obese and sick thousands of years ago as we are today, you probably would not be here to read this book. We would be long gone.

- We were not designed to be spending vast amounts of our income visiting doctors to get another Band-Aid for health problems and not getting down to fixing the real source of most of our ailments. Hint: It's inflammation.

- As you start to drop the sugar, grains, and bad fats, and embrace naturally sourced protein, organic fruits, vegetables, and an array of good fats, you will save so much money *not* going to the doctor and buying more pills that you *can* afford the pricier grass-fed meats more of the time.

Take Away Actions:

- Rome was not built in a day, but you *can* start to substitute another nutrient dense vegetable for the starchy component of your meals.

- Try breakfast without any breads—gluten free or not. A couple eggs, nitrate-free bacon, and a cup or more of veggies—maybe in an omelet—will hold you *longer* than the (SAD) Standard American Diet breakfast of toast, whole grain cereal, and orange juice.

They may be small, but the micro-nutrients that are discussed next are mighty! They help keep our engines running smoothly.

Small Wrenches—Micro-Nutrients and Water

We need those micro-nutrients to power-up the continuous body-wide chemical processes that facilitate proper functioning at every level! Like the job that is done when we grab a big wrench for a project to loosen or tighten large bolts, there is a place for the work load of small wrenches. No project is without a mixture of needing connectors with large and small bolts.

Our bodies are the same. Protein, good fats, and carbohydrates all have their role, but without the smaller connectors and tools to adjust them, we would not function well at all.

When I think of nutrient dense foods, I especially think of these micro-nutrients which are the vitamins and minerals that are so essential to keeping us going.

Each of the, approximately, 70 trillion cells in the human body function as a sort of a chemical reaction factory. Simply put, vitamins and minerals help drive those chemical reactions. We do not make our own vitamins and minerals. We must get them from our diet.

Human cell and tissue growth, development, and daily repair is driven by how our cells use the vitamins and minerals we eat. It is possible to be fed and *still* be malnourished. You will soon learn how certain foods we eat are contributing to this problem by damaging the lining of the small intestine to make nutrient absorption impossible.

To get the most from nutrient dense foods, we should strive for a variety in our foods. Rather than tracking down individual vitamins found in each vegetable, for instance, just go for a variety of colors. While a majority of our vegetables should be dark, leafy green, just don't think that kale and spinach are the only choices.

I have come to the conclusion from reading about different foods, that a balance is needed even in eating vegetables. The Yin and Yang of life, perhaps. Eating just one kind of green leafy vegetable can overload some things. Variety and balance are needed. If we rotate the color, we are rotating the nutrients we get from our food. So, mix it up! Different greens and an array of colorful vegetables to complete the picture.

There is no internal barometer for needing certain vitamins and minerals. We do not wake up in the morning thinking, "Hmm. I need some extra vitamin B3 and potassium today. We better have some turkey and sweet potatoes for dinner." Imbalances, diseases, and dis-ease are certain outcomes from vitamin and mineral deficiencies, but a day-to-day gauge is not available. We rely on our trusty brain to guide our choices.

Supplementation

Volumes have been written about supplementation. Everyone has an approach as to what is best and often that includes their own line of supplements. I am not going there. In addition to having nothing to sell, I do not feel qualified to make any recommendations myself.

In my reading, however, there are four or five supplements that keep coming up I will share with you. Among others, I am summarizing thoughts by Robb Wolf, Mark Sisson, and Dr. Tom O'Bryan.

Vitamin D

Number one on everyone's list is Vitamin D3, the "sunshine" vitamin. Our skin activates the manufacture of Vitamin D when the sun shines on it. Needless to say, people have gone overboard in sunning themselves, getting skin cancers at an alarming rate, and many have become disfigured from needed surgeries. Too many have died. Now most people slather themselves with SPF 50! Many in the Paleo community tout that a judicial sun exposure, coupled with an anti-inflammatory Paleo diet, allows for decreased bad side effects. You will have to work that all out with your dermatologist.

At any rate, increased indoor living, coupled with sunscreen usage, has greatly reduced our skin making Vitamin D the old fashioned way. A diet high in whole grains contributes to an inability to absorb Vitamin D. Even being obese or having a low intake of oily fish also hampers absorption of this vital nutrient.

Vitamin D is necessary for a host of processes and benefits including:

- Building stronger bones by helping bones absorb calcium

- Helping lower insulin resistance

- Decreasing auto-immune responses

- Assisting in fat metabolism

- Assists in lowering cancer rates

Since Vitamin D is the sunshine vitamin, I take it in the mornings with my meal. Work with your Doctor or Nutritionist about dosage.

Omega 3

Number two on everyone's list is Omega 3—the long chain fatty acid of EPA, eicosapentaenoic acid, and DHA, docosahexaenoic acid, which are found in wild fish and grass-fed meat. A summary of its benefits include:

- Decreasing cancer rates

- Decreasing auto-immune responses

- Increasing insulin sensitivity

- Decreasing insulin resistance

- Decreasing nerve degeneration processes

- Promotes healing of the gut

As I mention throughout this book, the Standard American Diet greatly promotes an imbalance between Omega 6 fatty acids and Omega 3 fatty acids. Even if you are eating a completely (as possible) non-inflammatory diet, some extra Omega 3s would probably be a help.

A personal quirk I would like to share is that both my husband and I noticed a little Omega 3 is good, but more is not necessarily better. When we took an additional fish oil supplement, we both noticed a drop in our blood pressures. My low blood pressure did not need any help at all, so I take just one fish oil capsule in the morning time when my activity will keep me pumped up. Another reason to work with your medical professional about all supplementations.

Prebiotics and Probiotics

All of our gut health, in addition to an intact lining, is dependent on the health and balance of the bacteria living inside of it.

Feeding the "good" bacteria is what prebiotics do. Prebiotics are carbohydrates that cannot be digested to be used by our own bodies, but serve as food for the bacteria, a.k.a. the probiotics. We supply prebiotics to our probiotics by eating foods such as asparagus, Jerusalem artichokes, bananas, onions, garlic, and honey.

Probiotics are found in natural, organic, fermented foods, and the live bacteria found in yogurt, kefir, kimchi, and kombucha.

This whole topic is about our microbiome—the microorganisms that populate our intestines. As our stress levels go up, the health of our microbiome goes down. Thus, we become wide open for opportunistic infections (infections that seize the opportunity of our weakened immune systems) and other diseases. In addition to stress factors, our microbiome is challenged by any sickness, travel with our being exposed to "foreign" bacteria, and the use of antibiotics which kills not only the "bad guys" but also the "good guys."

Many people supplement with probiotics. My understanding is to look for a variety of probiotics in your supplement. I use one with at least L. acidolphilus, B.longum, and B. bifidum. These are live bacterium, so dark bottles, far off expiration dates, and possibly cold storage are advantageous.

Magnesium

Often combined with calcium to facilitate calcium absorption, magnesium is a cofactor in bone formation. We get magnesium through eating dark green leafy vegetables. It is also absorbed through the skin in a relaxing, soaking bath with Epsom salts. Work with your health care professional about how to supplement with this vital nutrient.

One More Important Nutrient!

There is one nutrient, however, we DO have a sense for when we are running low! Any guesses? Water! Yes, lowly water. Mankind's first beverage after mother's milk. The beverage so many of us shun.

Water drinking should not have to be an acquired habit. We have been weened away from it by the sugar-pedaling industry of soft drinks. You will soon learn how sugary drinks **do not** quench a thirst. Instead, they make you want *more*! There's a science behind this I will reveal to you.

Learn to love water again. I have included a whole list of ideas in the Starter Recipe Chapter on how you can "tweak" plain water during your transition phase away from sodas and fruit juices. Flavor your own water, too! You are not looking for another way to ingest more chemicals and artificial colors found in commercially prepared flavored waters.

Take Away Thoughts:

- The basis for nutrient-dense food selections goes beyond seeking a balance of protein, fat, and carbohydrates. Vitamins and minerals actually drive the truck! Consider a variety of not only meats and fats, but also of the vast array of color and textures available in vegetables and fruits.

- Variety in foods is the spice of life and a keystone in getting balanced nutrition.

Take Away Actions:

- Go for the colors! All shades of green, orange, yellow, purple, pink, and red.

- Try featuring green veggies, plus at least one other color each meal.

- Make a contest with the kids to identify all of the colors and their sources.

Up next, how to maximize our success at improving our overall wellness by timing our changes and activities. Timing is everything.

RATCHETS AND TIMING LIGHTS FOR HABITS

"We are but a string of habits; each one a bead on the
necklace that is our day."
—Deidre Edwards

Knowledge of how habits work is the golden key to self-improvement.

Learning how to deconstruct the habit process is an invaluable tool.

After reading Alexandra Jamieson's blog on detoxifying the brain, and James Clear's free download called, "Transform Your Habits," I was able to break habits down to three steps. Understanding how habits work gave me the necessary knowledge and power to adjust them.

I will summarize the three steps to a habit that Alexandra Jamieson and James Clear wrote about:

1. The reminder or trigger that initiates the habit

2. The routine or action that is the habit, and

3. The reward or benefit of doing the habit

For example: I wanted to start the habit of drinking more water. Using my knowledge of how habits work made this happen. Here is what those three steps looked like:

1. I made the swishing out of my mouth first thing each morning to serve as the reminder/trigger that set me up for—

2. The routine/action of drinking one big 9-ounce glass of water which gives me—

3. The reward/benefit of doing something smart and positive for myself so early in the day which will help my digestion for hours to come.

This process makes me feel good about myself, gives me a sense of control over doing good things for my body, and instantly hydrates me. It may sound silly, but I like myself for doing such a kind thing for me. What a cool way to start a positive inner dialog each day!

We are now going to focus on the actual timing of creating better habits.

Tweaking 1.0—Small Changes Over Time

The thing to understand is, I was not forcing myself to start a big water drinking campaign. You know the scene: Standing at the kitchen sink several times a day, forcing yourself to chug this healthful glass of water? Tough to do, not pleasant, and doomed for failure. Why? A forced plunge into water drinking is drudgery. It commands vast reserves of willpower. Remember, the mind likes autopilot.

But you *can* drink ONE glass of water first thing each morning after you swish out your mouth. It is a point in the day when the palate and body enjoy the extra fluids. It's a small step. A small commitment. Easy to duplicate over time. Little "remembering" needed.

Instead, you are relying on the easy, natural trigger of swishing out your mouth which you *already* were doing. James Clear calls this "habit stacking," in which one new habit easily piggybacks onto an established habit. No rocking the boat. No willpower needed. Habit stacking.

Behold, you have the definition of what this whole Tool Kit is all about. Teensy, tiny "tweaks" to something you already are doing. Teensy, tiny tweaks that is easily repeatable. Consistent, daily tweaks over time will yield great big results.

Many people move on to drinking a second glass of water later on in their morning bathroom routine. I make it the last thing before I leave to head for the kitchen. Trigger: leaving the bathroom. Habit: Drinking a second glass of water. Benefit: "That deep down sense of satisfaction of a job well done!" (My favorite saying) Another benefit is my digestive process is ready to handle the day.

It has been proven time and again, grandiose changes do not work. Too much effort.

Use your understanding of how habits work and let that knowledge guide your tweaking. Call it the Law of Compound Interest, or "every journey starts with a single step," or call it, "Gradual and Consistent." Just chose to understand this key concept.

We all must understand it's the **tiny** steps that add up to **big** changes over time.

You probably will not see changes right away, but anything done consistently **will** yield great results over time.

You have to believe this basic law of the universe. Not understanding this basic law and not using it is why people fall out of starting new habits. In a world of instant gratification, we make two mistakes. One, as mentioned, we make too big of a goal or habit change which requires too much will power to sustain; and two, we want immediate results to push us forward. Do you desire a leaner body? A couple days of planks or crunches will *not* give you six-pack abs.

You *will* get a stronger sense of self-control and empowerment in just a few days of consistently doing a few minutes of these. Additionally, sticking to something gives such a sense of accomplishment. To me, this is priceless.

Second, after some more time, you will notice how easy these exercises have become. You will automatically look to increase the intensity (see the exercise section).

You *know*, as your calendar gets checked off every day, your exercise *will* make you more toned.

James Clear calls this the "Aggregation of Marginal Gains," in his blog entitled "Forget about Setting Goals." He writes about a football coach who led his team to phenomenal heights. He did not set goals of championships, but by set tiny goals of just 1% improvement.

Just like the idea of compound interest doubling a penny every day over the course of a month, a 1% gain does not look like much at the beginning. Have you ever studied the chart showing the growth of a single penny's investment that doubles each day for a month?

By day 10, that penny has grown to only $5.12. But by day 13, it is now $40.96. Then on day 18, it breaks into 4 figures at $1,310.72! Now the real visible growth starts! By day 28 that single penny has broken 7 figures at $1,342,177.28! If the month is not February, but maybe August, by day 31 there is $10,737,418.23!

With patience and persistence, that barely rising flat line on the chart of time will suddenly soar! Championships are won! Fortunes are made! Bodies are transformed!

The things you do for self-improvement must be repeatable. Small steps are repeatable. In whatever area you want to change or improve, find the **smallest** thing you can do, and repeat it each and every day.

Here is an example of how I applied this concept. I wanted to do a full body plank exercise for one minute. In February of 2015, I first cut the work load in half and the duration by 75%. I started with just half planks every day for 15 seconds. After a few days my plank lasted 30 seconds. Maybe a week later they were for 45 seconds. Finally, I conquered a half plank for 60 seconds.

I am now starting to also do full planks in March. As I write, those full planks are just 15 seconds. Sometimes I will do 2 - 15 second full body planks. But gradually, over time, I *will* ultimately do a full minute, full body plank. There is no doubt in my mind at all.

Take Away Thoughts:

- Like the proverbial drip of water cutting rock, mighty changes come from the accumulated effect of small actions.

- Think small, tiny goals.

- There are more habit stacking ideas throughout this book, so keep up the exploration of your Toolkit.

Take Away Actions:

- Explore "habit stacking" by drinking an extra glass of water first thing in the morning.

- If you can't wait, go to: https://booklaunch.io/deidre/toolkit-for-wellness to get your own idea list of easy tweaks as a part of your bonus material. I have compiled a list of easy tweaks you can incorporate into your daily routine. These "ETs" will give you a starting point in making small nudges to wellness. You will, no doubt, be inspired to come up with a few of your own! Please share your ideas with me at foodtalk4you@gmail.com so I can add them to the list for our community!

Tweaking 2.0—or, How to Get on a Roll, Stay There, and Gather Momentum

Once you have decided on one or two new habit tweaks, how do you keep it going day after day? How can you get on a roll and keep it positive, gathering momentum?

That leads me to habit tracking. I had seriously resisted doing this, but after reading many articles and books on habit formation and self-improvement, I can now heartily endorse the benefits of habit tracking. There are elaborate apps and programs out there for free and for purchase. I even made a sort of clumsy spread sheet when I started this (an Excel expert, I am not).

The spread sheet was, naturally, on my computer and had to be called up to be seen. Filling it out each day was another task in of itself. Once I left the screen, the visual reward of seeing my accomplishments was gone.

It is not insignificant that my excellent start to habit tweaking seriously slacked off once I dropped the spreadsheet and before I started putting check marks on a constantly visible calendar. For me, nothing trumps a good ole' paper calendar with check marks.

To make things easier, I have made a simple template for you to track your habits. Visit HERE (https://booklaunch.io/deidre/toolkit-for-wellness) to download your own Easy Tweaks Habit Calendar in your bonus material.

You will notice it is set up to track no more than three habits for reasons I will explain.

After ignoring advice to the contrary, I became frustrated trying to track 6 habit tweaks. It is best to limit working on just two, maybe three, priorities of tweaking a day. Any more, I just felt like I was living for a list, and that's not what this is about. We are talking about a journey and how a couple very small steps done every day can yield great results. We are after smooth and natural improvements, gradually made over time.

So, decorate the refrigerator or your bathroom mirror—where ever—with a simple calendar dedicated to your habit check marks. Being visible as a daily reminder and reward is important. It can also help with accountability and inspiration as the rest of your family sees your progress.

Don't start twenty new things to do...just two or three. After a month, add another item or two. Once an item becomes ingrained, it can be dropped from your tracker. That extra glass of water? I do not even think about doing it. It's on autopilot now. Doing my daily plank while the tea is brewing...still checking that one off. You'll know when you get to the point of "graduating" a habit off the list and into your daily autopilot hard drive.

By the end of the year, you will have mastered probably over twenty-four new habits...er...tweaks! When I started writing this *Toolkit for Wellness* in February 2015, my overfilled tracker looked like this:

1. Breathing mindfully followed by meditation and prayer

2. Reading the Bible

3. Exercising ten minutes—that includes those planks!

4. Writing, either this book, my blog at www.foodtalk4you.com, or both

5. Prepare for my *Designed for Health* class

It got the job done. Keeping a simple chart/log really pushed my motivation to fill it in each day; but a chart is not why I am doing this. I want to stay connected with myself and my Creator, to get into better shape, to excel as a writer, and to share what I know about wellness.

I cannot be a better writer if I do not write every day. I will not have a flat tummy or keep my strength and flexibility if I don't move.

By keeping track of my tweaks and commitments to myself, I feel so good when looking at the chart, I can hardly wait to do them again the next day. It's a win-win situation with charting. The habit is good and the reinforcement of seeing the chart is good, too! Charting just boosts the whole thing.

Another beauty of habit tracking is that it is a living document that changes as we go along. Today, as I finish the rough draft of this book in August 2015, my habits have become stacked and there are just two check offs covering several items. It looks like this:

1. A Series of Good Things

2. Writing

My "Series of Good Things" is how I start my day. It includes many of the ideas listed on the ETs (Easy Tweaks) List available free at: https://booklaunch.io/deidre/toolkit-for-wellness. It's just the easiest way I know to do everything I want to do in as short of a time as possible. I'll share some more about this in the next section which is about the timing of good habits.

Is there a better time to start them? Should you wait until the start of the week, month, or some other created starting point? Can't wait to share the answers with you in the next section!

Take Away Thoughts:

- Each time you put action to your daily tweaks for self-improvement, you gain momentum! Each day's small success builds on the next.

- Keeping a habit tracker is just another tool in your kit that helps create that environment for success.

- You have heard the adage, "The state of your bed is the state of your head"? I believe this. If you want to start a roll of good habits and get the gratification of positive tasks done, do not let this one escape you! Remember, it's mostly a brain thing. Right after that big glass of water or two first thing in the morning, keep that good thing going by making your bed. It takes—what—under sixty seconds to accomplish? I consider anything under the two-minute mark as something I will not put off. A two-minute or less task is insignificant and not something that merits procrastination or elimination. So, do it! One good thing may be an accident, but two? That's a pattern. Look out world! I'm coming!

Take Away Actions:

- Download your daily habit tracker template at: https://booklaunch.io/deidre/toolkit-for-wellness.

- Pick two or three small daily things to do that will improve yourself and your overall wellness

- Check off day one by doing them.

Timing Lights and a Two-Minute Countdown
When to start a new habit tweak.

Is there a better time of day to start a good habit? "NOW!" That's the answer!

We do not want to cause any delays in doing good things for ourselves. If we are going to rely on the concept of finding that perfect moment to do something, guess what? That perfect moment will never come. Opportunities for delay will arise every day. Once you resolve to do something, how can you ever justify **not** doing it?

A case in point. My husband's father mirrored most of the men (and some of the women) in the 1930s and 1940s; he smoked. At a point in his life when he was saved and joined the Church, he also resolved that he wanted to stop smoking. Always a frugal man, he bought in bulk. He was no different in buying cigarettes. Did he keep smoking until he was out of cigarettes? Of course not! If smoking was bad for his body tomorrow, then it was bad for his body today. Having nearly a case of cigarettes did not mean anything to him in the face of his decision! Out went the cigarettes that day, and he became a non-smoker.

Woody Allen once attributed his success to mostly one thing: "Showing up!" So, when is the best time? Now! Long before there ever was a Nike organization, my personal motto for getting through all the assignments for high school and college was, "Don't think about it. Just do it!"

Wringing your hands, obsessing with the enormity of the long range goal, and fretting over details are only delay tactics. Start, already.

Do your own very few, tiny, repeatable steps now. They may look small in the face of the ultimate goals you have, but do them—now—put this book down and do them. Then check them off your chart. Day one, done!

The best times of day for energy.

Studies and personal testimonies of countless people indicate, for most all of us, morning hours are best.

Immediately, I can hear you saying, "But I am just not a morning person!"

Let's just look back for a minute...way back, before electricity and for eons before that. For longer than we can imagine, our biology was set up and functioned to work in total sync with nature. We were designed that way. Our very hormones, which color our internal rhythms, were and *are* guided by the day/night cycles of nature. Hormones, which make us alert, ramped up in the day. Our activities happened in the daylight hours. As the natural light dimmed, activities slowed down, people stayed home and slept.

While not advocating ditching electricity, you have to appreciate that human kind has created an entirely different twist on the whole concept of day and night. As a result, huge advancements have happened, it's true; but those advancements are often at the life-shortening expense of people being out of sync with themselves. Hormone deregulation plays a huge role in many diseases. Then there is the "dis-ease" that many people feel. Not diseased, but not at ease within themselves. Using the tweaks and hints throughout this book will help you to rein in that feeling of dis-ease and strengthen your overall wellness.

The natural rhythms of the human body create clarity, focus, and energy in the morning hours. Use that biological truth to your advantage. Remember those 50-60,000 decisions we make all day long? By the end of the day, that desire for autopilot is strongest because of having to make all of those decisions. Tapping into creative juices and a fresh desire to move forward is best accomplished first thing in the day.

If you are waking up dragging your feet and yearning for that soft pillow, hang in there. You may need some of the 10 sleep hygiene hints in the next section. Improving your sleeping hours will play a key role in your ability to capture the natural energy you should have for the morning.

Exercising, for instance, is best done first thing in the day. Exercising sets up the body to continue burning calories long after the last push-up has been done, so starting the day with exercise just makes sense. With the body movement that exercise generates, all sorts of good things are happening to set us up for success. More rapid blood flow sends energizing nutrients and oxygen to the brain, muscles, and organs. Hormones to keep us alert are flowing. Our body is getting equipped to meet the day's demands. We become more focused. All systems go!

This getting "on the ready" is best done in the morning or before dinner, at least, because doing exercise after dinner would be counterintuitive to getting a good night's sleep. Of course, this is all predicated on the idea you are not involved in evening or night shift work. Whenever you rise, exercise is one of the best activities to prepare you for the active period of your day.

So, back to timing. When to do things? Clearly, food tweaks will happen when you eat; but other wellness habits need your priority—in the scheme of things. Personally, I prefer to start my day with my breathing, meditation, prayer, Bible reading, and 10 minutes of exercise because that really sets me up for a great day. But life happens. Many times it is mid to late afternoon when I can do what I want.

Oh, did you read that? What is the flaw in my thinking? Who is in control? I am. Because I am valuing my morning solitude even more, I am seeing an opportunity to make time for personal habit improvement by getting up thirty minutes earlier than I have been. I have read of countless others who are doing this already. There really is no other time of day to...start your day. However, there are times when it is mid-afternoon before I can do my personal habit improvement routine.

The bottom line is that I am doing it. Small changes. Every day. Over time, these tiny changes will add up. Guess what? I am now doing half planks for a minute, and full planks for 45 seconds now! Every day. Small changes. Over time. Make for great progress.

Take Away Thoughts:

- You know the expression, "the longest journey starts with a single step," is true. A simple-sounding truth, but so profound. Know that instant results are made only in commercials and most Hollywood films. Be more like "Rocky." Climb those steps EVERY day.

Take Away Actions:

- To ensure your success, set your daily goals so small that not doing them would be just crazy.

- Reward and motivate yourself with a simple system of habit tracking. Not only will you feel good about your daily accomplishments, but if others are around to see it, they can see your success and be inspired as well. Also, having your checkoffs in a public place is a great motivator, too.

- Get your copy of Easy Tweaks Ideas and your Habit Tracker Template at: https://booklaunch.io/deidre/toolkit-for-wellness.

- For beating procrastination, apply the two-minute rule. If something can be accomplished in two minutes or less, DO IT! This one idea has netted me so much success, a sense of great accomplishment, and power. It has also vanquished the burden of little tasks that had been hanging over my head, weighing me down, and cluttering my mind.

Now, put on your sleeping caps and learn about 10 actions you can take to set yourself up for a good night's rest.

Lights Out for Sleep

"Methought I heard a voice cry, "Sleep no more!
Macbeth does murder sleep"—the innocent sleep,
Sleep that knits up the raveled sleave of care,
The death of each day's life, sore labor's bath,
Balm of hurt minds, great nature's second course, Chief
nourisher in life's feast."
—William Shakespeare, *Macbeth*

Thank you, Mr. Shakespeare for so eloquently describing the purpose and the advantage of sleep!

Sleep: When the mind sorts through and processes a day's worth of endless stimulation.

Sleep: Which gives the weary body rest from its labors.

Sleep: Which helps us put the entire day in perspective.

Sleep: That which naturally follows the "first course" of having lived the day.

Sleep: Acknowledged as the part of the day that gives us the most nourishment.

But judging from study-after-study, we are becoming more like Macbeth who is doomed to no more restful, healing, or nourishing sleep. Not because we share Macbeth's troubles, but because...because... why?

We live in a world with constant stimulation available at our finger tips. Our lives are overscheduled. We seem unable to unplug and wind down at the end of the day. Then there are some people who try to believe that sleep is a gross waste of time, and they are above it all.

But look at the health status of the populace. Just today I read, if present rates of diabetes were to continue to grow unchecked, the medical expenses of diabetics alone will soon cost more than we are collecting from ALL taxes!

Why talk about Diabetes when I am supposed to be talking about sleep? Because missing even one night's adequate sleep can disrupt insulin levels. Being sleep deprived causes cravings for carbohydrates. Think about it. In the mornings when you are tired, are you grabbing carbohydrate laden "comfort" food such as a pastry or are you enjoying a protein-rich omelet? Not only will the pastry spike your blood sugar, but you will "crash" later spurring you to look for another "carb fix."

There are several simple steps to a more healthful sleep hygiene:

1. Sleep in the darkest possible environment. The glow of the LED dots on all of our devises throughout the house lights things up like a midway at night! Unplug your sleeping room. Blackout curtains do wonders. So do sleeping masks.

2. Reserve your sleeping room for sleep ... and sex ... but not for an office or movie theater. Walking into your sleeping room should signal your brain that restful sleep is on the way.

3. Try using just a nightlight lamp in the bathroom while you prepare for bed. Mine has a dark shade and really creates such a calming ambiance. The dimmer light starts the wind-down process by sending messages to the brain that night has come and sleep is near.

4. A relaxing bath with one cup of Epsom salts is a real relaxer and helps with magnesium levels. Soaking in a bathroom with a dim light...ahhh!

5. It sounds almost un-American, but disengage from those devises for at least an hour before bed. The light from the screens actually keeps our brains whirring

long after we have turned them off. They emit a blue light that is highly stimulating to the brain region telling us it is still day time so we should be ready to "Go!"

6. Keep your sleeping room comfortably cool.

7. Studies have shown, keeping the last meal three hours from bedtime helps, not only digestion, but sleeping processes. Having lived with a lifetime of bedtime snacks, I am gradually working up to just two hours. Rome wasn't built in a day, but eating right before bed is a recipe for gastric reflux and poor sleep. Look for a snack high in good fats and protein. Check out the Starter Recipe Chapter.

8. Steer clear of "night caps," or excessive drinking, at dinner time. True, alcohol relaxes... initially, but later its effects can actually keep you awake.

9. Before dimming the lights for your going-to-bed-routine, make several entries in your gratitude journal to point your thoughts to the positive and reflective.

10. Before or right after lying down, take five or more deep, slow, calming breaths.

A note about restless legs. I have learned from a friend's chiropractor how to rid myself of those twitches by doing a very simple exercise that sort of gets that extra energy right out of my legs. This routine is the first step I take earlier in the evening to get ready for bed each night. No drugs to take either! Remember, exercise is stimulating, so this is best done way before bedtime.

Here's the trick: Lie on your back and peddle those legs like a bicycle. I do one hundred "pedals," followed by rolling to my side to do ten leg lifts, rolling on the other side to do ten more. Following those straight body leg lifts, I usually also do ten leg lifts on each side with my top leg at ninety degrees to my body. Often, I will follow this with 50-100 more bicycle pedals on my back. There's no way my legs will keep me awake after that! ZZZ!

Take Away Thoughts:

- Respect the very human need for sleep. Our ancient ancestors slept in the deepest of dark with only the moon and stars for light. We need to create sleeping spaces that closely reflect that.

Take Away Actions:

- Disengage from electronics at least an hour before sleep.

- Develop a sleep hygiene routine that contributes to your mental, physical, spiritual wind-down with dim lighting, relaxing mineral baths, and a cool sleeping room.

- Note: Keep regular sleeping hours all week long. Binge sleeping on the weekend causes a disruption to your sleep pattern and takes several days to adjust back to normal hours.

Next, there is a tool you can throw out of your toolkit right now. What is it?

Volt Meter Not Included

One thing *not* included in your *Toolkit for Wellness* is a calorie counter. You know, those endless lists with how many calories in every food type there is, as in green beans: raw, steamed, boiled, roasted, sauteed in oil, sauteed in butter, canned, frozen---well, you can definitely "let it go!"

Why? Because calorie counting is based upon numbers—quantity—not quality. Number comparisons mean if you can have 500 calories for lunch, then a Snickers bar, just 1 ounce of potato chips, and a very small banana would do the job! Any real nutrition there? Enough to keep you going for hours? Keep you at the top of your mental capacities? *No.*

I would refer you to Jonathan Bailor's book, *The Calorie Myth,* for a very detailed presentation on why we do not need to be beating ourselves up about calories. Suffice to say, we need to be looking at the **quality** of what we are putting in our bodies and not so much the *quantity*.

Additionally, protein and fat are very satisfying and filling. A meal with protein and good fats is hard to over-consume because of the high satiety factor. Whereas, a meal with hefty amounts of starchy carbohydrates may have fewer calories, but it's hard to satisfy the hunger factor, and often results in overeating or needing to eat again sooner.

Certainly, a person could gain all kinds of weight blindly overeating even quality foods; but on the average, studies have shown eating extra calories of proper quality food (soon to be defined) will assist in effortless weight loss. Let's face it, minding calories is a recipe for frustration, defeat, and failure. We have probably all done it. It's such a colossal waste of time.

Take Away Thoughts:

- We will be mindful, not of calories, but of nutrient density. We will be looking at cause and effect—natural bodily responses to different types of food.

Take Away Action:

- You can throw away any calorie counting lists or books!

There are some major topics yet to be explored that will rock your understanding about food and how it is affecting you. Pieces of the puzzle will start to come together with a deeper understanding of inflammation and how something most people tout as 'good' is actually very 'bad' for you. Conventional wisdom definitely comes up short!

GETTING DOWN TO BRASS TACKS

So, where does this all leave us? Let's look at what has been covered so far:

You have all the tools for wellness already. You just need a bit of guidance on how to successfully use them to give you maximum benefits.

It all starts with a thought: You learned techniques to be more mindful, centered, and calm. You have practiced mindful breathing and are, hopefully, doing that throughout your day in order to get your body into a perfect, balanced metabolic state to greet the day, start a project, or unwind from the day's activities.

You have learned that changing your health status for the better does not require drastic life changes. In fact, you have seen how little tweaks are the absolute best way to move forward, accomplish long-term goals, or get better at any task. Keep doing the little tweaks every day. They are to be so small and insignificant that they do not require will power; they require consistency. Remember, they are so easy to do, they would be equally easy not to do, too! Just *know* you are on the right path and even though there are no evident changes today, there *will* be changes over time.

You have expanded upon the tools available for your improved sleep. You have learned that sleep is necessary, not only for daily healing, repair, and thought processing, but is also vital for maintaining a natural weight and eating pattern that promotes health.

Are you drinking that extra glass of water first thing in the morning right after you swish out the cobwebs? Yes? Great!

You have taken a mini-course in the anatomy and physiology of the digestive system and certainly must be impressed with how wonderfully intricate your "second brain" is to the smooth functioning of your body.

The basic elements all food is broken down into have been explained, and you have been made aware of the implications of eating the (SAD) Standard American Diet versus eating a diet of naturally sourced food—basically food with no ingredient labels.

Did I say that all—yes all, disease is rooted, at least in part, to inflammation? Guess what? We are totally in control of the inflammatory processes in our bodies. Yes. It's a matter of choice—oh, there goes that brain thing—yes, choice. If you truly want those blood sugars to be stable, if you really want to have more energy, if you are determined to get a 'happy belly' again, then make some tiny, repeatable tweaks to your life and see how you feel in 30-60 days.

Very soon, you will read about "ditching" certain foods, but we are not approaching this with a hang-dog face. Rather, we are opening a door to neat things that you *can* eat, enjoy, and delight in! There is a whole world of really great food out there that is not laced with sugar, wheat, and preservatives. Really!

Now, we are left with needing to have a clearer picture of what to eat and how to exercise. Let's start with food. No actually, let's start with an understanding about inflammation and then grains. Making food selections is locked into understanding what those choices will net us. What is their bottom line and why?

Inflammation

Apologies for having bantered this word around so much without really explaining it.

Inflammation can be a beautiful thing, an intricate process our immune system initiates when potentially deadly invaders, (bacteria and viruses), break through our number one defense: our intact skin and the linings of our body cavities.

This is great when we cut or scrape ourselves. As the torn edges of the capillaries begin sending out signals that start the clotting cascade to stop the bleeding of our wound, the immune system is sending special fighters to wage war on any invaders and clean up the debris.

We are all familiar with this scene. Our cut or scrape becomes red, hot, swollen, and painful. This is our body in one of its finest hours, protecting us from ultimate harm! But there are times when this intricate system gets confused and attacks our own bodies, thinking our *own* cells are the bad guys. That describes autoimmune disease.

In the next section, you will learn how glutens can cause a physical breakdown of the lining of the small intestine. This breakdown is known as intestinal permeability or, in layman's term, "leaky gut." Globs of incompletely digested proteins, and any toxins we may consume, get absorbed directly into the blood stream. While floating all over the body, they are recognized as invaders.

War ensues! Anywhere and everywhere, affecting the proper functioning of tissues and organs. Migraines, foggy brain,

ADHD, irritable bowel, bad skin, achy joints from arthritis, heart disease, and hormone irregularities, you name it.

With the understanding that every disease known to us is somehow rooted in the inflammatory process, is it such a novel idea to perhaps eat a diet that does not trigger body-wide inflammation?

Take Away Thoughts:

- Inflammation can be a friend or a foe.

- We have to help our body by not laying the ground work for body-wide or systemic inflammation.

Take Away Actions:

- We can choose foods that are non-inflammatory and can actually calm down inflammation.

Coming up: How to find those healing foods.

Glutens, and Lectins, and Phytates, Oh My!

To quote Judy Garland from The Wizard of Oz, "I don't like this forest—it's dark and creepy!" "Do you suppose we might meet any wild animals?" To which the Tin Man replies, "Mostly lions and tigers and bears!"

"Lion, and tigers, and bears, oh my!"

When you delve into the forest of so-called whole grain goodness, it's a clear case of: "Glutens, and lectins, and phytates, oh my!"

While Judy and the gang became fast friends with the bashful lion, we are in no way friends with glutens, lectins, and phytates.

Why? What are they anyway?

Well, going back to a better understanding how things work, let's look at the nature of what we eat.

All living things work very hard to protect their own life. Animals run, jump, fly away, and if caught, claw, squirt toxins, sting, and bite to stay alive.

What's a plant going to do? Clearly not jump out of the ground and run!

Plants protect their precious seeds with coverings that are hard to penetrate, like nuts and their shells. Some fruits have noxious skin such as mangoes. Grains protect their seeds with toxic anti-nutrients: glutens, lectins, and phytates.

Let's look at each of these to see what is happening when we eat grains.

You may have heard of gluten. There are more and more foods in the market being labeled "gluten free."

Briefly, gluten is a protein found in wheat, barley, and rye grains. Gluten, the lectins, and phytates found in other grains, can affect a couple factors in the integrity of the structure and proper functioning of the lining of the small intestine.

Remember Dr. O'Bryan's analogy of the fuzzy, shag carpet structure of the small intestine lining? The shag carpet structures need to be maintained for proper absorption of nutrients. They can become damaged, bent, crushed even, which renders them useless in nutrient absorption. To keep his carpet analogy going, in the presence of glutens, we now have Berber carpet.

If that's not disastrous enough, the integrity of the junctions holding the individual cells of the small intestine lining together is compromised and the intestine becomes "leaky"— also known as intestinal permeability. This is where systemic inflammation and autoimmune issues start.

Inflammatory processes are good if we have cut our finger. Temporary inflammation helps with healing the cut; but body-wide, chronic inflammation leads to auto-immune issues and disease.

All humans produce a protein called zonulin when gluten is consumed. People with Celiac Disease produce way too much. The excess zonulin causes the junctions between the cells lining the small intestine to open up, allowing toxins, and clumps of gluten molecules to get through which are then absorbed into the blood stream.

Imagine molecules of protein escaping from being absorbed for use and instead, are floating around and being seen as foreign invaders. Our bodies will naturally mount an immune response which is what starts the inflammatory process I have outlined previously. Where ever this immune response happens is where trouble happens, pick an organ, any organ; pick a body system, any body system.

Researchers are saying more and more, the bedrock of most all disease is auto-immune in nature. The gluten found in wheat, barley, and rye (and the lectins and phytates in other grains and nuts) are what serve as a launching pad for auto-immune and inflammatory diseases. This is why the signs and symptoms of any level of gluten sensitivity are so broad.

To summarize an article of Dr. Tom O'Bryan's, "The Gut-Disease Connection," from May 8, 2014, the first step in the development of autoimmune disease is leaky gut. In the event we can reverse the leaky gut, the possibility of shutting off the autoimmune response becomes real.

Lectins bind to our insulin receptors, our intestines, and also seem to cause problems with our responding to the leptin hormone I mentioned earlier—that's one of the hormones that tells us we are full and satisfied.

Finally, phytates round out this nightmarish scenario by making the minerals we eat bio-unavailable for absorption. This natural human reaction to phytates means you will not get the minerals you need from the food you eat.

Is that dark, creepy forest of whole gain goodness looking even creepier yet? Can you connect these dots to the ills we see all around us?

Why are we becoming a nation of people who are obese, diabetic, weak boned, anemic, tired, and head-achy, with ADHD in our children, and victim to mounting auto-immune diseases and Alzheimer's? Has our DNA broken down?

Science is getting smarter but we are getting sicker! What's wrong with this picture?

1% of us are allergic to gluten in a drastic way and symptoms of Celiac Disease, as it is called, can manifest fairly early in life. There are Celiacs who have no digestive issues; and there are non-Celiacs who are gluten intolerant with *plenty* of digestive issues. I have read recent articles stating there are some people on the gluten sensitivity spectrum who are only reactive to wheat. But sometimes it can take decades before the relenting damage reaches the threshold of causing life-altering disability. In fact, I want to share Bob's story with you right now so you can appreciate what gluten overload, good stress, and bad stress can do to an adult body.

> Bob's Story: After coming to America at age 17 from Asia, Bob enjoyed a totally American life, immersed in its culture, including the Standard American Diet. Fast forward to Bob at age 70, as he and his wife enjoy a summer trip to Germany and Austria. The good stress of a vacation in Europe is easily off-set by enjoying the cuisine-du-jour, which certainly includes fabulous German and Austrian pastries, breads, and bakery goodies three times a day. Ah! Very exciting times! Maybe not enough sleep, but plenty of pictures and good memories.

> Before they returned home that same month, Bob was experiencing symptoms of a cold, some diarrhea (traveler's diarrhea?), and decreased appetite. Had Bob picked up some kind of virus? Okay, many travelers pick something up, nothing serious. They were back home the next month, in July, and Bob became very, very sick with nausea, vomiting, and diarrhea every day. Needless to say this trim man of 125 pounds was rapidly losing weight. The doctors ordered a host of tests, especially for cancer; but they all came back clear. One doctor called this

"mysterious" and wondered if he had, indeed, picked up something exotic in Europe.

Add to this mix the stress of moving to another state to be closer to family, leaving behind fabulous friends and a strong church community. Needless to say, Bob got worse. By March the following year, Bob and his doctors were convinced he was going to die. He was down to 79 pounds. In a last ditch effort, his test results were forwarded to Massachusetts' General Hospital for further analysis. Finally an answer was coming!

Bob had become so allergic to gluten, he was "one notch away" from being a person with full blown Celiac Disease. He had become gluten intolerant. It took eight months to finally get a diagnosis. Eight months of suffering.

Four months later, still on a gluten-free diet, Bob is now back up to 112 pounds and feeling better each day. It took a couple weeks for him to see any changes for the better, but improvements are happening all along as his body heals.

None of us are immune to the onslaught of forces that create some degree of gluten sensitivity.

Nearly 30% of us are non-Celiac, but test positive for antibodies that indicate the body is at war with itself in some way or the other when gluten is ingested.

In all of my readings, I have never heard of a single person who has not felt better after they stopped eating all forms of gluten. They felt better, they often lost weight, their brains were clearer thinking, their aches and pains lessened, their arthritis improved, their energy levels improved, and their bellies were happy. Truly the list goes on and on. But your grandma lived to be 102 and she ate bread all of the time? Well, Grandma's wheat was not the wheat we are eating today. The dwarf wheat grown now is especially high in gluten.

Grandma did not grow up with the food pyramid touting whole grains as the foundation of a healthy diet either. She ate lots of vegetables, farm fresh eggs, and meat—and she walked everywhere. Remember that story of her two-mile trek to school in the winter?

What is one to do? Give gluten-free a real try for 30-60 days; and if your symptoms improve, great! If you improve somewhat, but still have some level of dis-ease, then expand your eliminations to include *all* grains (rice, corn, oats, etc.). Once you are normalized, try reintroducing non-wheat grains, one at a time, and note your body's response. Everyone is unique. Maybe you can eat a bowl of oatmeal or a serving of rice.

Take Away Thoughts:

- Aside from adding to a starchy carbohydrate-laden diet, which causes great swings in blood sugar levels and promotes fat storage, grain consumption presents *other* problems that contribute to destruction of the small intestine lining and can lead to systemic and chronic inflammation.

- Eliminating grains is a must for some of us, not only in terms of gluten reactions as in Celiac Disease, but also in terms of the lectins and phytates tearing up the small intestine lining.

- Some people are successful at reintroducing select grains such as white rice or corn after they have healed themselves through total grain elimination.

Take Away Actions:

- Give healing a chance! For just thirty days, eliminate all gluten and just see how improved you feel. I predict you will start feeling better after just 7 days.

Stay tuned and keep reading. I will show you just how easy this is going to be. There's guidance for every step of the way. Choose to help yourself to improved wellness.

What's in a Name?

We are fond of names and labels, so it is valuable before moving on to first understand what some of the food and dietary approaches mean.

The Standard American Diet (SAD) is loosely based on the old Food Pyramid laced with the effects of highly-commercialized food "products." The Food Pyramid boasts whole grain goodness as its broad "eat mostly this" base, and vilifies fats as sure killers. It is interesting to note, since the inception of the Food Pyramid model, obesity and diabetes began to skyrocket. Mere co-incidence?

Well, think about it. Grains are broken down and processed as the carbohydrates they are. Carbohydrates are broken down by the digestive system into simple sugars. ALL carbs are broken down into SUGAR (glucose or fructose molecules). So, be it a whole wheat bagel or a piece of frosted birthday cake, the end result is sugar! To transport that sugar to body cells, insulin is needed. Any sugar fuel not needed at that time is stored as fat.

While eating the carb-centric diet as outlined in the Food Pyramid, Americans were requiring their bodies to produce more and more insulin. After a while, being awash in insulin, our bodies become resistant to the effect of insulin—sort of ignoring it.

However, our cells were starving for the sugar fuel. We were still hungry, so we ate more whole grains. Can you see the vicious cycle this was, and is, making? Gaining weight and becoming diabetic. There's a term for that: diabesity.

Insulin is known as the hormone of fat storage. Eating carbohydrates causes a need, not only for insulin production, but *receptivity* to it effects. As one who often suffered from frequent low blood sugar crashes, I mistakenly tried to "fix" things by eating carbs. True enough, my blood sugar would go up, but as all of that insulin took effect, my blood sugar crashed again. Little did I know at the time, cutting back on the (starchy) whole grain carbs with each meal, would have normalized my blood sugar! I certainly know that now. I can return to low blood sugar crashes quite easily if I heavily re-introduce starchy carbs—even gluten-free ones—into my meals. Instead, I rely on protein and good quality fats, along with low-glycemic, colorful veggies and fruits to keep me on an even blood sugar keel.

A word or two about food products. You know them. If given the long list of their ingredients, you could never guess what they were. A lot of money goes, not only into the production of those items, but extensive money and research goes into *selling* them to us. It's all about money, making money, and making more money. Our health is not even on their list of concerns. Making a profit *is* the list.

Eating Clean or Clean Foods ...

... is all about eating unprocessed food, as close to the original source or form as possible. This type of eating eliminates the highly processed oils, food products, and "Frankenfoods," such as prepackaged meals and junk food, (chips, cookies, frozen pizza, Pop-Tarts) in favor of real, identifiable food (apples, carrots, steak, tomatoes, and kale....You get the idea). This might also be referred to as whole foods. Mind you, this also contains whole grains......

Gluten Free ...

... eating eliminates the inflammatory proteins found in wheat, barley, and rye. Using simple gluten-free alternatives for common starchy foods such as bread, crackers, and cookies will address the gluten-sensitivity but not necessarily address maintaining balanced blood sugars or weight loss. Gluten is also found in condiments; thus, label reading is needed.

Paleo, Paleolithic, Ancestral Eating or the "Caveman Diet" ...

... are all terms used to describe how our ancient ancestors ate prior to the advent of agriculture. It could be described as clean eating or whole foods, but without gluten, most other grains, legumes, soy, and using dairy only if it is from pasture-raised animals and if dairy is personally tolerated. Refined sugar is out. The elimination of all grains (in addition to those with gluten) would mean no rice or corn because of other elements—phytates—that can cause inflammatory processes.

Take Away Thoughts:

- What is in a name? It is certainly good to understand some general terms; yet, there are no reporters interviewing us about what label we have or are calling our diet. I mean, I just grab my meat, veggies, and fruit and go to the checkout line! Paying is a must—not labeling.

Take Away Actions:

- Look around at the other grocery carts and the people who push them. I can predict how they will look (healthy glow, haggard, overweight, hyper) just by looking at the contents of their carts. I can even spot those who are trying their best for their families but failing miserably because their food choices are based on faulty thinking—Their carts are full of whole grain goodness in everything...even their junk food.

What's coming up next is a description of what our goal is in terms of food selection. Understanding the general terminology first was important so you can understand where our blueprint is headed.

BLUEPRINT FOR 'THE PLAN'

Now we are ready for 'The Plan'!

You probably wanted to read about this on page one, but everything is a process. There was so much more to this picture than just what to eat for dinner. Engaging the brain was foremost in understanding we are actually in control. The hypnosis of the TV commercials and misinformation have deluded most of us. We have been on an initial journey into empowerment. Knowledge *is* power. Without overwhelming you with deep, detailed science, my goal has been to give you a basic understanding that will help you put everything together.

Looking at foods that heal and protect our wondrous digestive system and promote over-all health is what seems to be the key. That's why you were first given a tour around the small intestine. You spent some time learning about how protein, fat, and carbohydrates are broken down from what we eat and what elements are essential. You learned how stress and sleep deprivation affects what we eat and how it changes our body chemistry. Now you know how inflammation running amok sets us up for body-wide immune responses which lead to auto-immune diseases. Finally, there were the goblins in the forest of whole grain goodness which were revealed to be not good at all.

Labels are just labels. An anti-inflammatory diet is certainly going to be our starting point for discussion. There are all levels of what would constitute an anti-inflammatory diet because each one of us is unique. Truly, you won't really know what you need until you sort of wipe the slate clean. Really clean. Discover how you feel with all of the bad players off of the court and you can feel the new, yet original, you.

You certainly must know there is room for improvement if you are reading this book. Others of us may not even be aware there is something better out there—some level of healthful glowing they did not know existed. But it *is* there for each of us! We were designed to feel vibrant, alive, and full of energy! It's hard to know you are missing that "sparkle," when perhaps you never had it or it was so long ago you have forgotten.

Based on what we have covered, doing away with inflammatory triggers and eating foods that nurture our anti-inflammatory balance is where improved health can be discovered. You can call this Paleo if you wish; but the bottom line to me is that it is anti-inflammatory.

You May Need an Elimination Diet First

Using your doctor as a guide, if you *know* you have serious issues, an elimination diet is the way to jump in. I am all about gradual and consistent, tweaking habits and all, but if you are desperate to "do anything" to feel better, an elimination diet is the best way to wipe the slate very clean. This is usually in the form of a 10-day detox. Many people have resources for this such as Dr. Mark Hyman in his book, *10-Day Sugar Detox*, in which he will hold your hand and guide you through this process. The "Whole 30 Plan" is a very popular approach to regular body resetting and wiping the slate clean. Even those who are already eating a nutrient-dense, non-inflammatory diet usually do The Whole 30 once a year to "reset." I am not trying to replicate that process here; but I will give you some information about what elimination diets are about.

Each of us is unique. Each of us has a different starting point; and many food problems are interlinked. Wiping the slate clean and reintroducing foods has yielded great results in fine-tuning what works for our own needs. Such a diet is caffeine-free, sugar-free, alcohol-free, grain-free, and dairy-free. It is created from whole food—not prepackaged or prepared foods—because of the long and often-toxic ingredient list.

Even then, certain carbohydrates from various vegetables and fruits can cause problems, and some people do better on an SCD diet or Specific Carbohydrate Diet. If you have been on an elimination diet for a couple weeks and are still having health issues that show no sign of improvement, then I suggest Jordan Reasoner and Steve Wright's website SCDLifestyle.com to get more help. Also, seek to establish a relationship with a physician and a nutritionist who support functional medicine. A SCD diet is gluten free, sugar free, starch free, and totally unprocessed. Like many of us have had to do, Jordan and Steve had to find and learn their own path in the wilderness of misinformation to save their own health. Their mission is to help people by sharing their wisdom through personal experience.

Our Approach, Plan, and Take Away Thoughts:

- Our plan's goal it to be as non-inflammatory as possible, but be as nutrient-dense as possible. Such an eating plan is a Paleo approach, which is inherently anti-inflammatory.

- Keeping the lining of the small intestine intact and happy is our goal. That lining is *one cell thick*! Its cells are intricate, tough, and highly specialized! Our unifying, mind-set shift exercise earlier on reinforced that holy bond with our body. That relationship is a commitment to listen and protect. We will listen, respond, and protect our bodies as they listen, respond, and protect us.

- By eating an anti-inflammatory diet, we will be working in sync with our bodies, going in the same direction toward balance and daily wellness.

Follow along as each element is discussed and helpful tips and tools are shared to ease you into the ultimate eating plan. The eating plan we were designed for. The *original* eating plan. The plan that does not lead to auto-immune diseases. Get ready! Here we go!

Measuring Tape

Does your food measure up in terms of nutrient density?

More than anything, looking at the nutrient density and value, or answering the question, "What's in it for me?" will revolutionize what you put into your body. What happens to an automobile if the wrong kind of fuel is put in it? It. Does. Not.

Work. It may become permanently damaged. We wouldn't even think of doing that on purpose. A car can be one of our biggest investments. We would never want to jeopardize its proper functioning.

One of the first things we do in getting a new car is ask what kind of fuel it uses. So, why do people think their beautifully and wonderfully made, intricate, precise, and you-only-get-one-to-a-lifetime body can function as planned when feeding it...I'll be nice......junk?

For eons, humankind has been eating real food, close to its original source. What makes us think that we can put highly-refined, partially-hydrogenated oils into our "engines" and expect them to work smoothly? How many food dyes, chemicals, or pesticides does it take to poison us? Who can expect vibrant health when eating food so far removed from its original source that it no longer bears any resemblance to the real thing?

Our bodies just have not adapted to use all that is being put in them today. Around the world, as nations have financially grown in the global economy, people consider having Western fast food eateries as a "badge of honor" for having "made it." They long to see the "Golden Arches" along their thorough fares. However, as they switch from the whole food/real food diets they were used to with no particular resulting health problems, they suddenly develop great upswings in heart disease, cancers, diabetes, obesity, and Alzheimer's. Diseases related to highly-processed western diets.

Straying away from whole food and relying on food that causes inflammation, creates what I call "negative nutrition." Every day, our bodies need fuel for activities, healing, and constant repair. Damaging the small intestine damages the ability to absorb even the good stuff. Pretty soon, the body is running on a deficit. No energy for life. No building blocks for repairs. Building up toxins. Misplaced immune response. Wrong fuel. Bad outcomes.

Nutrient density is paramount after the question of inflammation has been handled. Using a mental image of a measuring tape, measure the nutrient density of what you are feeding your body:

"Is this meal going to promote the smooth functioning of my body and nourish it/fuel it for today's activities?"

"Is this meal full of glutens, lectins, and phytates that will not only block nutrient absorption, but will also do physical damage to my body?"

"Will my second brain and the center of my immune system be damaged and send confusing signals to my body?"

Take Away Thoughts:

- Remember the references to a very small action repeated over time always yielding big results? The same principle applies to negative actions. One burger with fries and a soda may make no particular change to your ultimate health. It's just once. But repeated over time...? You got it. It's a downhill trend and a slippery slope, indeed.

- Thing is, doing that one, teensy good thing for yourself is just as easy *not* to do. It's a teensy thing. The teensy thing could even be small and insignificant as to be viewed as boring.

- That glass of water, for instance. Easy to do. Just as easy *not* to do.

- What will make *you* a winner at wellness is *understanding*. While you may not be able to appreciate big changes today if you choose a green salad with grilled chicken, you know that over time...it most definitely will. We may justify a slip here and there, but would we want our bodies to *ever* function at less than *their* best? We want to function and feel our best *all* of the time. Negative nutrition will not put us on top of our game.

- *There will be bad outcomes to wrong fuel.*

Take Away Actions:

- Measure *all* of what you eat. Empty calories? Lots of chemicals?

- Accept the responsibility that *you* are in control and *always* have a choice. Honor that pact you have with your body each and every day.

Guess what? As I type this in April 2015, I can do a full body plank for one full minute. No kidding! Little actions over time yield great results.

Now you will be digging into a big first step. It's an important one that will color everything else. Read on.

Ditch the Sugar

If you are just getting started in cleaning up what you eat, start ditching the sugar first. It is so liberating to not pine for another sugar "hit". So many people are trying to do this by simply switching to non-caloric sweeteners, but that seems wrong on multiple levels. How natural is it?

Additionally, there are so many studies showing people using artificial sweeteners actually overeat. See, the artificial sweetener is telling the brain that sugar is on the way. When blood sugar levels don't go up, the brain sends the signal to eat in order to raise the blood sugar. Guess you can't fool Mother Nature!

There's Stevia and the like but to me, that's still nurturing a sweet tooth *if* you maintain starch consumption that has been 'cleansed' by Stevia. If we are just talking about your morning coffee, fine. I often have a small amount of sugar in my coffee, too. It's there, but it is not enough to give me a blood sugar spike that throws me off balance.

We are surrounded in the stores with all kinds of packaged, sugary wonders, but just looking at the ingredient list of an Oreo cookie sends shivers down my spine. Talk about "edible food-like substances"! Isn't there supposed to be a natural instinct to protect ourselves? Turning away from poison should not be that difficult, folks.

Given the Standard American Diet, however, it *is* hard. Very hard. Why? Because it is laden with sugar and grains in the form of breads, pastries, pastas, cookies, and cakes. Sugar is a particularly addictive form of carbohydrate. It lights up the OPIATE receptors in the brain. Really! Our brains naturally respond: "Bring it on!" This brain reaction, by the way, also happens with starchy carbohydrates. You can see why this combination can be a devil to stop.

But I am a firm believer that knowledge brings enlightenment, and that enlightenment should mold our actions. If we 'learn' things but do not change our behavior, then we really haven't learned anything at all, you know? Let's learn some more cool stuff you may not have known about sugar that has made giving it up difficult. Yes, aside from actually being addictive in the brain, there's more.

Sugar does not quench thirst or hunger. The same way cigarette manufacturers secretly ramped up the nicotine content of their products to make them even more addictive so smokers would be customers for life, those *same* manufacturers are now involved in the manufacture of packaged foods. They employ people to find that "sweet point" for each food product they produce. Can you find some kind of pre-fab food product with no sugar in it? If those companies can't hook us on their nicotine, they are hooking us with sugar. In fact, they are taking it a step further by hooking us on high-fructose corn syrup, which is by far cheaper for the manufacturer and much more damaging to the human body.

Please remember this: sugar does not satisfy. A soda will *not* quench your thirst. It was not designed to. Do you remember Biology class?

How certain solutions would:

1. draw water out of a cell,

2. cause the cell to absorb the solution, or

3. be neutral to a cell?

Put that cell in a sugar solution and it will *lose* water. Sugar. Will. Not. Quench. Manufacturers *know* this. They are counting on us to be ignorant and addicted.

It seems to be a no-brainer, looking at the terrible upswing of obesity, diabetes, ADHD, Alzheimer's, and other auto-immune diseases, something has changed. We just haven't gotten cleverer at diagnosing patients. We are *creating* those patients by how we have changed eating.

Without getting very technical and scientific, let me summarize what I have read from a dozen books and numerous articles on line: Sugar is inflammatory, not to mention addictive, in a very real way.

We just reviewed all of that inflammation information but I want to add just a bit more science-y stuff about cholesterol and triglycerides.

"Wait!" you say. "That's fat stuff. You were talking about sugar."

Those two topics are more related than you think. Just hang on and I will clear things up for you.

But first, one resource I just have to share with you is Mark Sisson's, *"The Primal Blueprint."* If you are looking for deep scientific explanations, he's the man. He clearly has thoroughly researched every detail, and his book is a cornerstone for understanding clean living and eating. I highly recommend it.

On page 80 in the hardback version, he starts explaining about cholesterol's role in our good health, where it is created, how it is transported throughout our body, and much, much more. I will endeavor to boil his insight down to the bare essentials.

Oh, and the sugar thing, I'll be getting back to that very soon.

Cholesterol is so important to our overall health processes and actual structural integrity that our liver makes it. Because it is a fat molecule and is transported in our watery blood stream, it needs a carrier. (Remember how fat and water do not mix?)

The carriers for cholesterol are lipoproteins such as LDL, HDL, (those you may have heard of), and VLDL (which may be new to you).

VLDLs are made in the liver when there are high levels of triglycerides present in the blood stream from the types of food eaten. VLDLs carry mostly triglycerides and a bit of cholesterol to fat and muscle cells where it downloads the triglycerides but retains the cholesterol. Empty of their triglyceride loads, these VLDLs convert to either fluffy (harmless) LDLs or small, dense (harmful) LDLs.

What drives whether they become harmless or harmful? The general level of high blood triglycerides causes the body to convert the VLDL into small, dense LDL, which is harmful. Why are small, dense particles of LDL so bad? They get trapped between the cells lining the arteries, get oxidized, become inflamed, and lead to plaque formation and heart disease.

What can be done to lower triglyceride blood levels?

Good question! NOW we get back to the sugar thing. See, I promised.

A high-carbohydrate diet, which inherently causes an excessive production of insulin, drives the conversion of those excessive carbohydrates into triglyceride fat particles! Insulin drives the production of triglycerides.

You have already learned sugar is a carbohydrate. The Standard American Diet is bursting at the seams with an average of 150-170 pounds of sugar per person, per year. That's not counting the starches and whole grains some would have us eat. You remember all of those carbohydrates are broken down into... that's right... sugar molecules called glucose.

What is needed to transport glucose? Insulin! Right!

Are the light bulbs starting to flash? A high carbohydrate diet needs lots of insulin, and excessive insulin production drives the conversion of excessively eaten carbohydrates into fat particles called triglycerides. BAM!

Take Away Thoughts:

- So, yes, ditch as much sugar as you can.

- Controlling bad forms of cholesterol can be done naturally, through food choices.

- Choose health. Knowledge often comes with a burden of making new choices. Now you know better. Now you can move forward with conviction that comes through knowledge.

Take Away Actions:

- Oh, that's the second part of this section. Keep reading so you can tame that sugar tiger and banish him back to a jungle far, far away.

How to Ditch Most of the Sugar

Noticed I switched from "Ditch the Sugar" to "Ditch Most of the Sugar"? This is not intended to be a slight of hand trick or a bait and switch scheme. It is reality... and a plea for sanity. The goal is not to eliminate every molecule of sugar from our diet. We should not become maniacal super-sleuths banning a dollop of ketchup on a hamburger patty. We need to just be mindful of where a whole plateful of sugar will take our body.

Depending upon the severity of your sugar or "sweet taste" addiction, there are basically two paths to take. I added the words "sweet taste" to the mix because so many of us are still under the gravitational pull of needing everything tasting sweet. Most all prepared and commercial food products rely on the sometimes subtle sweetness of sugar to keep us coming back for more. Even some home cooks have added sugar to the veggies to help lure the little ones to eat their nightly portion. So, to varying degrees, we all have some kind of a sugar habit to kick. You are not alone. Help is here.

Good books have been written about this, saying that sweet cravings can actually be due to calcium and magnesium deficiencies compounded by a possible zinc deficiency which robs people of tasting food very well at all. Check out Mira and Jason Carlton's book, *Macronutrient Miracle* for a whole new approach to understanding cravings.

There are two ways to ditch most of the sugar: cold turkey or gradual and consistent. Sort of depends on if you are the type to jump in the pool or to gradually lower yourself into the cool water. They both get the job done.

Cold turkey.

Many have done this. It can be very hard, if not hand-wringing hard, for a few days. There can be actual withdrawal symptoms of general malaise to headaches. Then it becomes just 'hard'. Life still seems to have no spark. Toward the end of the first week or so, your taste buds start to wake up and notice other flavors more.

Your diet, while going cold turkey, should contain so much good protein and veggies, (both cooked and raw), that there is no room to even put dessert. Snacks of nuts, seeds, avocado, and some fresh fruit should be handy if needed. Active, athletic members of your family can still eat healthy starches found in plantains and sweet potatoes. Make sure to rely on the sweet spices listed in Foods, Cooking, and Condiments 101; and beef up savory and spicy flavorings to your dishes to distract you from the lack of "sweet."

Once you have gone through that first week, each day becomes better and brighter. You will be learning of new flavors you may not have noticed before. Your blood sugar levels should be rock solid without the sugar-induced swings. You will actually feel better, with more energy and vibrancy. Your head will be thinking clearer.

The best part? The *absolute best* part? That comes when you taste something sweet and you instinctively respond, "Ick!" because the sweetness is so over-whelming.

Gradual and Consistent is another fine approach.

I did this with soda consumption at work. Soda was not a big part of my life... ever; but I picked up the habit of having it with some meals and as a treat sometimes after a hard day of teaching. I just started either buying those little mini-cans or I would buy a full sized beverage from the teacher's lounge *only* if I could share it with someone. I liked sharing because I could maybe help inspire someone else to cut down with me.

At restaurant meals with my husband, I would have water and just take a few sips of his soda. My husband still chooses to drink soda on occasion. That's his choice. I then converted to unsweetened tea with a splash of sweet tea. Gradually, I have totally kicked all soda and sweet tea.

Kicking the sweet of cakes, cookies, and the like, came two-fold for me. Because gluten intolerance can be hereditary, I stopped eating gluten because our daughter has Celiac Disease. Additionally, because of my knowledge and understanding of glutens, lectins, and phytates, (oh, my!), I did not want baked goods made with wheat, barley, or rye flours.

Most commercially available or restaurant baked goods are full of gluten. BAM! A lot less sugar consumption, right there.

Take Away Thoughts:

- Except for eating honey, ancient people lived and thrived without being awash in any kind of added sugar. Berries, fruits, and coconuts were it. That's how our digestive systems were designed to work. We just have not evolved enough to handle the 150-pound annual sugar consumption most Americans are doing. In fact, such eating patterns are spelling extinction of the human race through obesity and diabetes! There *is* a choice.

- When your taste buds can come out of their sweetness stupor and appreciate subtle natural sweetness in coconut, berries, and spices, a whole new world opens up.

- Whether you go cold turkey off of all sources of added sugars, or go more gradual and consistent, ditching the added sugar is one of the biggest gifts you can give yourself.

Take Away Actions:

- Cut down or cut out. Sugar is usually linked to starchy foodstuffs anyway, so you will be doing yourself a *double* favor.

The sluggishness sugar induces—not to mention the weight gain and off-balance blood sugar levels—is really making me reconsider how I will be approaching "holiday baking" this year. Gluten-free or not, there's always a price to pay. Check out the Special Times Chapter to see how to tweak special occasion foods.

So, what's left to eat? Oh, lots and lots, my dears. Keep reading.

Meat, Meat, Meat and Other Protein Must-Haves

Every meal should have a significant protein component. There are no essential nutrients in carbohydrates, but there are essential nutrients in protein.

Because variety is the spice of life, learning how to switch up protein sources lends excitement and interest in food.

In the "Perfect Plate" section, you will see eggs do not have to be the sole source of protein every morning. While eggs are pretty versatile and can result in a wide array of dishes, eggs every day can get boring. Boring could lead to wandering into realms of sugar and starch. We choose to not go there, right?

Speaking of eggs, however, are you a part of the trend? So many people are raising their own chickens for fresh eggs. If you have not done this yourself, maybe you can connect with someone in the area or at the farmer's market for some fabulous free-range eggs from happy chickens. Needless to say, they are better for us and have a superior balance of fats than eggs from mass producers. Even those eggs in the store that declare they are cage-free just means there's an open door somewhere to leave the building... If only they could find it through the thousands of other hens.

Pasture-raised or grass-fed animals not only have a happier life and are not filled with stress hormones, antibiotics, and added hormones in their muscles, but their fat profile is better than feed-lot raised animals. They have higher levels of Omega 3 fatty acids. Whenever possible, grass-fed is the best.

While grabbing a pasture-raised slab of beef and throwing it on the grill is delicious, aim for variety of meat sources to gain the nutrients, flavor, and balances of other proteins. Leaner cuts of pork, lamb, and other game are perfect.

Ground meats can be combined to vary and enhance flavor while lowering the overall fat content. Add ground turkey or chicken to change up hamburgers or meat loaves usually made just from beef. If shopping for meatballs, search out the gluten-free versions. Continue to read the package label to make sure you are getting whole food ingredients without added sugar.

Most recipes for meatballs and meatloaf all call for bread as a softening ingredient. When making these dishes, just switch to gluten-free bread crumbs! If you plan your time well, preparing a large batch of homemade meatballs on "cooking day" could help you out for weeks to come.

You can change up the presentation to match your mood: Italian style in a tomato sauce could go on "Zoodles" (see recipe section), Asian style with gluten-free and soy-free alternates to soy sauce (see Condiments, Herbs, and Flavor Enhancers), paired with Cashew Gravy (see recipe), or sliced on an open-faced, gluten-free bun.

A discussion about protein sources cannot leave out fish and seafood. Fresh caught fish can enhance our intake of Omega 3 fatty acids. Such cold water varieties of fish include: Sardines, herring, anchovies, salmon, trout, tuna, and mackerel. Seafood sources include: Oysters, mussels, shrimp, clams, crab, and lobster.

I have read some research that states the development of the human brain was in direct proportion to early man's access to the Omega 3 fatty acids from ocean fish and seafood! Who are we to turn away from such a power source for our brains?

Farm-raised fish live a life similar to feed-lot animals. The fish are jammed-packed into an area too small to live a natural life, resulting in elevated stress hormones for the fish and a heightened absorption of toxins. Additionally, they are being fed a diet that contains chemicals and antibiotics. Farm raised fish also have much lower levels of the beneficial Omega 3 fatty acids.

Chia, flax, and hemp can also be added to smoothies, puddings and fruit (see recipes), and sprinkled over salads or added to baked goods to boost nutrition. All great sources of Omega 3 fatty acids, they also add fiber and 2-10 grams of protein per serving!

A note about hemp. One of my Designed for Health participants asked if he would get a positive drug test from adding hemp hearts to his diet. The answer is no. The hemp grown in Canada (our source in the U.S.A.) is tested and controlled for THC, or Tetrahydrocannabinol, levels. If dietary hemp is your *only* source of THC, then you will not test positive based upon what I read from several sources including PubMed.gov. Best to check with your employer, however.

Nuts are another alternate source of protein. A small handful of activated or sprouted nuts is an ideal serving size and an excellent snack. Fiber, good fats, protein, and lots of flavor...Nuts are fun to add to any meal for a nutritional plus.

You may be asking about soy. So many think turning away from meat and switching to tofu and soy beans is going to be a healthy thing. I used to drink smoothies made from soy protein. I never could put my finger on it, but they just never felt "right" to my insides. Since then, I have learned that unfermented soy is actually estrogenic, meaning it has compounds called phytoestrogens that mimic estrogen.

Consuming a lot of soy products, according to my readings, can create hormone imbalances for both men and women.

As Corey Pemberton wrote in an article for Paleohacks.com on August 17, 2015, estrogen mimicking can cause low testosterone and low sperm count in men and has been linked to increased risk for breast cancer and menstrual cycle irregularities in women. He also quotes studies that show soy can disrupt the proper functioning of the thyroid gland, causing symptoms of low thyroid. The thyroid issues resolve when the consumption of soy products is stopped.

Additionally, unfermented soy is a grain which puts it in the category of foods that can cause inflammation. Inflammation is the key factor in destroying not only small intestine health but the health of our whole body through initiating disease.

Remember those mineral absorption-blocking lectins present in all grains? Well, soy products have those unfriendly lectins, too. Those lectins, as you recall, disrupt the, "I'm full" hormone, thus contributing to increased hunger. Increased hunger leads to weight gain, which leads to obesity, which leads to Diabetes. These factors all work in lock-step to our detriment... *if* we choose to consume them.

The health of our gut is the seat of our whole body's health. Soy is just another item that starts those dominoes falling.

Take Away Thoughts:

- So many I know who think they are taking a healthier, maybe a more humane, approach to protein by not eating meats are still suffering from migraines, belly issues, weight control, and other concerns. I just do not think we were designed to not eat animals. Certainly, the historical record supports that.

- What we *can* do is support the ethical and humane treatment of the animals we do eat. Not just because it is the right or nice thing to do—which it is—but because 75% of the antibiotics produced in the U.S. goes to the feedlot animals we eat. Antibiotic resistance is not just because we may be relying on them too much to treat people, but because we are eating them all day long if we are eating feedlot meats.

- Then there are the hormones. We are eating those feedlot hormones ourselves. Not to mention the stress hormones that permeate the animals systems because of such an unnatural and stressful life. We have enough stress in our own bodies. We do not need to feed ourselves stressed meats.

Take Away Actions:

- If at all possible, support and benefit from pastured, grass-fed meats.

- Whatever the source, include protein with every meal. Rely on the protein, good fats, and the non-starchy veggies to get you through the day!

Okay. We have a fillet of baked, wild salmon seasoned with garlic, lemon, dill, pastured butter, kosher salt, and pepper. What to eat with it? Let's explore those possibilities as we, "Embrace Vegetables and Fruits in Season."

Embrace Vegetables and Fruits in Season

What does "in season" have to do with anything? We can eat strawberries twelve months out of the year. Who cares?

Following local seasonal food is like heeding to our own circadian rhythm. It's like stepping in time with nature, swimming along with the current. Sure, it's fun to fix an amazing spinach salad in December with fresh imported berries and blue cheese as a treat, but following seasonal food is answering deep, natural, and cyclical nutritional needs that come with the seasons.

There's a reason we eat apples in the colder months. Maybe the type of fiber in the apple helps brush out harmful viruses and bacteria. Maybe the apple's fiber is better suited to our slower physical pace during indoor months so our bowels can be regular. Whatever it is, there is a Master Plan with the changing seasons, and I like to go along with it.

The best part of seasonal fruits and vegetables is that it means we can buy local, farm fresh produce. Whenever possible, shopping at the produce stands and farmer's markets is always going to yield fresher, more nutrient-dense food. Even the grocery stores are getting produce sections featuring regional farmers from within the state.

Are you like me? Do you taste your vegetables first when you start eating? By varying the cooking oils, methods, and seasonings, veggies can be the centerpiece of taste, flavor, texture, and color on your plate.

Maybe you were subjected to bland, limp, lifeless vegetables as a child. Canned or cooked-to-death veggies, rings the death knell for many a child's dinnertime! For generations, children have discovered all kinds of creative ways to hide or give away their lackluster vegetables.

Banish those days! Not by giving up on vegetables, but by giving them their just due and cooking them in a way that opens up their aromas, flavors, and nutritional benefits. There's a whole bright, colorful, and flavorful world out there in properly prepared vegetables.

In the section entitled, "Never Boil Again!" you will learn why boiling is not necessary or desired. I don't think I have ever met a vegetable that cannot be gently sautéed, and possibly followed by a light steaming with little to no extra water to finish.

I can't wait for you to see some easy ways to prepare vegetables that will enhance your diet and health by providing you with the nutrients you need to thrive. That will all be in the Starter Recipe Chapter coming up.

Let's talk about getting those vegetables and fruits in season at your grocery store—sort of "Shopping 101" or "How to Avoid the Pitfalls of a Grocery Store."

In general, the perimeter of most grocery stores is where the fresh food is. The canned and packaged foods are in the interior of most store layouts. Armed with that, there is just one basic rule to follow:

Buy the bulk of your foods on the perimeter of the store. Period.

On the perimeter, you will find the fresh vegetables and fruits, meats, and eggs. That is what you need, everything else should just be condiments, coffee and tea.

There are just a few canned things that I use: tomato paste, diced tomatoes, diced green chilies, olives, full-fat coconut cream, pineapple cubes in their own juice, unsweetened applesauce, and boxes of organic, and free-range chicken broth. That's pretty much it.

Even the gluten-free bread I buy is in the frozen section on the perimeter! Sometimes there is an occasional purchase of some gluten-free crackers or noodles, but the interior of the store hardly ever sees me.

Buy fresh and cook fresh. The time spent in food prep is negligible compared to the incredible benefits. So if you can't get to a produce stand or the farmer's market, there is a way to shop at a grocery store and still get what is good for you.

Fruits in season are a delightful component of a rich, colorful, varied, and nutrient-dense diet. All types of berries are at the top of my personal list because of their high levels of vitamins, excellent antioxidants, and phytochemicals, which help with maintaining a healthful, youthful body, and mind. Berries are also lower on the glycemic scale, meaning they do not impart a big sugar "hit."

Tropical fruits and oranges are higher on the glycemic scale, but can be enjoyed in moderation, for sure. If weight loss is a main health goal, stay clear of daily fruit consumption and steer more towards the blueberries.

Cherries are also one of the super-fruits. They have been shown to have compounds that help with arthritis, blood pressure, gout, and with the addition of having melatonin, cherries help with sleep.

Check out the chia seed fruit pudding/jam and my, "Fruit with Benefits," recipes to see how to ramp-up fruit goodness.

A note about frozen food. Perhaps you, too, have read the many articles pointing out frozen fruits and veggies are actually fresher because they are picked at their peak and quickly frozen. So true. Fresh grocery store fruits and veggies have generally spent a very long time in transit and were picked before they were ripe.

I am just concerned that the frozen food people are pushing prepackaged frozen vegetables in steam-able pouches and are often pre-sauced with a long list of chemical ingredients. First of all, cooking in plastic is a major no-go because of the transfer of toxins to the food. We just shouldn't do it. Second, the merits of fresh frozen veggies can go south very quickly if you are adding a long list of chemical ingredients to them. Just be careful what you choose and how you choose to cook those frozen vegetables.

Take Away Thoughts:

- You are not alone if fresh vegetables are a little foreign to you. I grew up with plenty of canned vegetables, too. Canned vegetables were just a staple. No wonder green beans weren't thrilling. Unless, of course, they were in a casserole with *canned* cream of mushroom soup topped with deep fried in "Franken-oil" onion rings coated with who knows what. What a hit of salt, chemicals, and partially-hydrogenated junk oils!

- Fortunately, there is a better way as presented in this book. Congratulations on choosing to seek nutrient-dense and non-inflammatory foods to boost your wellness and fulfill your promise to your belly.

Take Away Actions:

- Shop the perimeter of your grocery store.

- Shop fresh fruits and veggies at local produce stands and farmer's markets.

- When choosing frozen, aim for plain versions you can enhance with whole ingredients on your own.

- Do not microwave, bake, or boil in plastic pouches!

Ready for a snack? There are some tricks to learn about a common "good" snack. I'll show you, next.

Nuts and Bolts

Nuts and seeds can be a powerful source of nutrients in a small package. But maybe you have noticed they can be a source of digestive aggravation as well. Why is this?

Consider two things:

1. Were those nuts and seeds "activated" or "sprouted"? Meaning, were those raw nuts and seeds first soaked and dehydrated? Activating or sprouting nuts and seeds is absolutely key in making them digestive friendly. Remember "glutens, lectins and phytates, oh my!"?

While nuts and seeds can be an excellent source of protein and good fats (omega 3s), they also have phytic acid (phytates) in their coverings. These phytates are the storage form of phosphorus and they bind to the minerals we ingest making them not absorbable by our digestive tract—meaning, we will not absorb zinc, calcium, magnesium, or the like.

You may also have experienced the very unpleasant feeling of undigested nuts scraping through you in the "going to the bathroom" process. That's because the nuts and seeds have enzyme inhibitors that prevent premature sprouting. These enzyme inhibitors are difficult to digest. This can be the reason we often have unhappy bellies or even bowels after eating nuts that have not had the enzymes and phytates neutralized.

We humans lack the enzyme necessary to neutralize the phytates on our own. To mitigate these problems, soaking and dehydrating these nuts and seeds neutralizes the phytates for us.

The recipe section will take you step-by-step through the neutralizing, activating, or sprouting process. No special equipment is needed other than some large trays and an oven. If you do have a dehydrator, that's great, too.

2. Were those nuts or seeds processed in some kind of "Franken-fat"? You know, those commercial oils, long removed from their original form, which are prepared in high heat and chemically treated? Those partially hydrogenated and trans-fat oils may enhance the flavor and shelf-life of commercially prepared foods, but they play havoc with our bodies.

When you activate or sprout your own raw nuts and seeds, enhance their flavors with fresh coconut, olive, or avocado oils and spices. You know you are getting the best. Your tummy and whole body will thank you!

Taste Test

Make your own taste test. Set some raw nuts aside, soak, and dehydrate the rest. Try a raw nut, and then try one you have activated. No comparison. Light! Flavorful! Crunchy! They just feel good to eat! Then take any commercially prepared nuts you may still have around and try one. Then try one of your activated nuts. One is heavy, the other is light.

Squirrels don't care! Give them the leftover commercially prepared nuts and save the good stuff for your family.

Don't forget to check out the recipe section for complete directions for easily creating the best nuts ever. There's also a recipe for some great trail mix and even a recipe for Cashew Gravy.

Take Away Thoughts:

- It is good to note coconuts are NOT nuts. Yay! If you have bad reactions to tree nuts, the wonderful world of coconut flavor, taste, and texture is still open to you.

- Peanuts are NOT nuts either! They are a legume and belong in the creepy forest of "Glutens, lectins, and phytates, oh my!"

Take Away Actions:

- Activated or sprouted nuts are so worth any effort it takes to get them. Try it once and you will be hooked for life. Finally, a nut that digests well. Hooray!

We just have to get a better understanding of oils. Fat gives us great taste, flavor, and is filling, but there are definitely ones we should *not* be using!

Good Fats and Oils

There was a time when we were lead to believe that "good" and "fat" could not co-exist in the same thought except, fat tastes good. "Fats" was a four letter word that spelled doom.

Actually, science proved that saturated fat COULD exist in a health-promoting diet a long time ago, but that information was cleverly hidden in plain sight for decades. A nutrition scientist, Ancel Keys, successfully and selectively manipulated data to support his anti-saturated fat theme back in the early 1950s. In actuality, that same data, taken as a whole and not hand-picked, proved quite the opposite.

Denise Minger's in-depth analysis of the hype that laid the groundwork for what we were trained to regard as a healthy diet is all explained in her revealing book, *Death by Food Pyramid*. She reveals the full data of study-after-study, along with the politics—yes, *politics*—that was and is driving our view of food. Another case of "follow the money" and the power. Nothing to do with the actual health of the populace.

She cites a 2011 review in *The Netherlands Journal of Medicine* in which the paper's authors suggest, "Dietary saturated fat—while not a health-harming entity in and of itself—may become problematic if it's dumped on top of a soup of inflammation and excess carbohydrate."

That's exactly what we are talking about in *Toolkit for Wellness*. The bigger picture is, judicious use of healthy fats *along with* an anti-inflammatory diet with modest starch intake, is healthy and desired!

Robb Wolf in *Paleo Solution,* and Mark Sisson in *Primal Blueprint,* do an amazing job of explaining all things technical and scientific regarding fats. I will boil the topic down to what fats we should be eating and cooking with to build an anti-inflammatory diet for wellness.

The world of fat is divided into saturated fats, monounsaturated fatty acids, and polyunsaturated fatty acids.

Saturated Fats

Coconut oil is special in the category of saturated fats. It consists of medium-chain fatty acids which have been shown to be anti-inflammatory and protective of the immune process. Coconut oil is linked to being protective from degenerative diseases such as Alzheimer's. The bacteria-killing property of coconut is well established. The breakdown of coconut oil in the body also leads to more efficient metabolism.

Coconut oil is highly saturated which confers to it a high level of stability in terms of shelf-life and its abilities to withstand high-cooking temperatures

Also, coconut oil is a key ingredient in my own skin moisturizer. Mixing equal amounts of coconut oil into my hand and body cream, I have been able to lock in moisture without a greasy feel. I have seen advanced dry skin in others return to normal, non-flaky skin with the addition of coconut oil to daily moisturizing.

The benefits of coconut's properties can be enjoyed many ways:

- Oil: which is solid at room temperature and liquid when heated,

- Coconut flour: for cooking and baking,

- Unsweetened coconut flakes: which are a great addition to trail mix and baked goods,

- Coconut milk and coconut cream from full-fat coconut milk: which can become like whipped cream, and

- Coconut water: which can be an excellent base for smoothies or as a carbohydrate beverage after vigorous sports.

Coconut oil can be a real flavor treat as you change up oil choices. I do not use it every day, but more as a flavor enhancer to pan frying French toast or pancakes for that added sweet factor.

Real, pastured butter from "happy cows" brings out the wonderfulness of steamed vegetables like nothing else. Ghee (clarified butter) made from pastured butter is excellent for higher heat cooking. Pastured or grass-fed butter has a better ratio of Omega 3 to Omega 6 fats. It also contains more nutrients, namely CLA—conjugated linoleic acid—which can be protective against cancer.

Monounsaturated Fatty Acids

The category of fats called MUFAs, or monounsaturated fatty acids, are considered to be "heart healthy." MUFAs include:

- Olive oil: not the inexpensive kind available in plastic jugs at big box stores, but the Extra Virgin Olive Oils grown from organic sources and packaged in dark glass bottles. Excellent for salad dressings and low-heat cooking. The whole Mediterranean Diet concept is all about healthy olive oil. Just about any dark green leafy vegetable sauteed in olive oil will give you a one-two punch of great, nutrient-dense eating.

- Avocado: both as a food and as an oil. Looking for a snack before dinner? Nothing like a quarter of an avocado sliced with lemon pepper on top. Avocado is a very satiating food with a smooth texture and mild flavor. And, who could turn away from guacamole? As a cooking oil, avocado oil has a high smoke point and is great for stir fry cooking.

- Dark Chocolate: also on the MUFA band-wagon, this gem is a delight for most of us. For some people, the "dark" part initially is not as fun. See, we are not talking about Snickers Bars here, we are talking 70% or darker chocolate. For me, dark chocolate was an acquired taste, but since I dropped the addicting sweetness of sugar-laden foods, dark chocolate became a favorite.

Not only does dark chocolate satisfy a deep desire for seductive taste bud satisfaction, it has a host of benefits. It has fiber and a host of minerals including iron, magnesium, copper, manganese, potassium, phosphorous, zinc, and selenium. And that's not all! Dark chocolate is loaded with compounds that function as anti-oxidants. Check out my recipe for "Magic Mousse".

- Nuts and seeds: offer a wide range of nutrient bonuses in fiber, protein, fat, vitamins, and minerals. Each kind of nut and seed has its own profile of benefits ranging from gut health, brain power, anti-cancer benefits, anti-inflammatory properties, to improved artery health. Almonds have the highest protein count, macadamia nuts have the highest MUFA profile, and walnuts have a lot of Omega 3s, but are high in Omega 6 as well.

Bottom line: Nuts are more of an adjunct to our dietary selections, not the main course. A handful is the appropriate quantity for a healthful, filling, and lasting snack or garnish. Just make sure they are "sprouted or activated" prior to eating and *not* commercially processed in bad oils.

Polyunsaturated Fatty Acids

Polyunsaturated Fatty Acids, or PUFAs, can be divided into the Omega 3s and Omega 6s.

There are good ones and bad ones, largely based on their origin and level of processing, with many, including corn oil and canola oil, coming from grains. Need I say more? Plus, they are highly processed. Some of the bad oils are the PUFAs sprung on us by the government and commercial forces back in the day they were telling us saturated fat was bad. Just about *all* processed food is made with these cheaper oils that do our bodies harm.

Another reason they are harmful is, they are unbalanced with an excess of Omega 6 fatty acids which, in abundance, are very pro-inflammatory. These Omega 6 PUFA oils include safflower, corn, cottonseed, peanut, soybean, and canola oils. Highly-refined. Not good.

To reiterate, great sources of Omega 3s include salmon, mackerel, sardines, walnuts, and chia, hemp and flax seeds.

Take Away Thoughts:

- Fat satisfies!

- Fat imparts great flavors!

- It's hard to over eat fat because it fills you up so well. Carbohydrates, on the other hand, are easy to overeat; even though carbs have fewer calories per gram, we tend to overeat them, thus consuming more calories overall.

Take Away Actions:

- Enjoy the natural moderation of consuming good fats.

- Favor olives and olive oil, avocados and avocado oil, and Omega 3-rich foods.

- Make sure your saturated fat sources are from optimum sources such as organic and minimally processed coconut oil, and grass fed or pastured butter.

We have all of the pieces:

- Good meat

- Great selection of colorful vegetables

- Good fats

Let's put them on a plate to see what this looks like!

The Perfect Plate

How about a template for good nutrition? Wouldn't it be easier if you could have a meal-to-meal, plate-to-plate guide for a nutritionally dense meal? Breakfast, lunch, and dinner? Well, I've got you covered!

Everything you are learning in *Toolkit for Wellness* is about helping you equip yourself for success in reaching a higher level of wellness. The ideas of:

1. engaging your power of choice,

2. breaking down big goals into consistently actionable steps, and

3. understanding how different foods break down to benefit or harm the body

4. have brought you to wanting to do what's right for your body with food.

While I call this The Perfect Plate, it is more of an ideal, something to aim for. Sometimes, we just have to make do. That's okay. An overriding principle that must be maintained is *not* to strive for perfection. The hazards of seeking perfection in eating are covered in the last chapter called, "Have Fun, Not Ulcers!" What most people use as a guide is the 80-20 rule. The 80-20 rule takes out the pain of pressuring yourself to do it all right all of the time. Let's look at the practical application of the 80-20 rule.

The 80-20 Rule

Widely embraced as the most livable model for life-long eating health, the 80-20 Rule works.

Simply put, 80% of the time you are eating nutrient dense food that:

1. causes no inflammatory response,

2. is free from chemicals,

3. is as close to the source as possible (not highly processed), and

4. was humanely raised.

80% of the time.

In the remaining 20% of the time you are *not*, however, throwing yourself under a donut delivery truck! Instead, you are *mindfully* flexing your food criteria to something that is *still* good for you. An example would be adding gluten-free bread as a small part of your breakfast. The bread may be gluten-free, but it still could command a starch hit if other grains were used. That's okay because you are not relying on gluten-free bread as a part of every meal that day.

Some of us may even entertain a little gluten *if* we are not supersensitive or reactive to it on an occasional special event but certainly not every day. Just understanding that gluten can cause a serious reaction for up to two-weeks after ingestion, makes me think twice about having any at all. Sometimes that bite of crusty French bread is worth a cramping to the gut later...sometimes it's not.

If you are Celiac or otherwise highly reactive, there is **no such thing** as "a little bit of gluten". One can liken such thinking to "being a little pregnant." There is no such thing!

Or maybe, you have come across a great gluten-free dessert recipe but it still has a big sugar hit to it. I often cut those sugars down to the bare minimum, and then make the dessert. Remember, sharing those special treats is a good way to make sure you do not eat the entire pie or cake by yourself.

Honestly, once I lost the sugar addiction, sweet things became a turn off. Ewe...too sweet. My *Designed for Health* students have echoed that experience. It is amazing how our taste buds can begin tasting something other than sweetness once we derail that sugar train.

If your 20% ends up being a plunge into the deep end of a pool of Kool-Aid or Sally's 14 layer death-by-chocolate torte, then "coming back" to the comfort of the 80% might have its challenges. Remember how sugar lights up those opiate receptors?! Take it easy, "A little dab will do ya'!"

With the 80-20 rule tucked under our belts, let's see how the protein, good fats, and non-starchy vegetables look on the plate!

The Perfect Plate looks as follows for all meals:

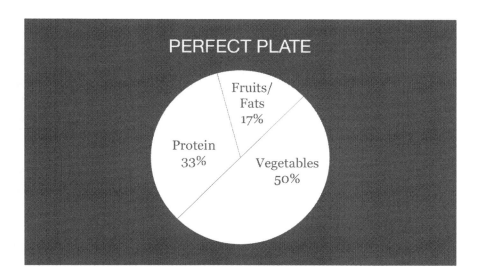

Half of the Perfect Plate is non-starchy vegetables. That would include anything green, colorful assortments of summer squash, zucchini, peppers, carrots, and the onion family.

There's more to green veggies than broccoli and spinach. Take another look at the vegetable section in your store. In my mind's eye, I am scanning the greens in my local Harris Teeter. I see Brussels sprouts, three kinds of Swiss Chard, cabbage, large and small Bok Choy, Broccolini, Broccoli Rabini, green beans, okra, collards, kale, turnip greens, leeks, asparagus … I know I have missed many others.

In the winter months, I will supplement a serving of greens with a serving of baked winter squash…sans cupfuls of brown sugar but flavored with pastured butter, nuts (see how to sprout your own nuts in the Starter Recipe section), maybe some seeds, and "sweet spices" such as cinnamon.

Two-thirds of the remaining half plate is reserved for the best lean protein you can find and afford as already discussed in the previous meat section.

The remaining section of the Perfect Plate is reserved for good fats sources and fruit.

A Starting point for The Perfect Breakfast Plate or Glass

If cooking from scratch:

- 2 slices of nitrate-free bacon or sausage
- 2 eggs
- Assorted veggies—green ones, at least

Cooked separately or together, this will last for hours. Sometimes after I plate my eggs and bacon, I will grab an enormous handful or two of baby spinach, baby kale, or both, and toss them into the same pan with a little extra oil, if needed, such as ghee, pastured butter, olive, or avocado oil. Stir leaves, and in a minute or two, they will turn into a small serving of greens. Top off with a pinch of salt, maybe a small splash of toasted sesame oil. Good stuff! Cook everything together and call it a fritata, or create an omelet. Mushrooms? Bell peppers? Green onions? It's all good!

Just today, I worked with what was in the refrigerator for breakfast. No bacon or even any leftover meat, so I sautéed some onion and a clove of garlic until well done. Then I added the last handful of spinach, stirred up two eggs with a cooking spoonful of full fat coconut milk, salt, and pepper. Poured the eggs on top of the veggies, added 1/4 cup of sprouted pumpkin seeds, and cooked it. Amazing!

For an added boost, sprinkle hemp hearts over the top for additional protein and Omega 3s.

Fan of pancakes? How about pancakes without the starch from flour? Check out the recipe for Paleo Pancakes in the recipe section.

Fan of waffles? Got you covered with a recipe you can check out on the blog by Paleo Parents with their Frozen Waffle recipe, which is a favorite of ours.

In a rush but still want to eat? Try my recipe for "Breakfast Cookies" that can adapt to what's in your cupboard.

Spread Justin's All-Natural Chocolate Hazelnut Butter Blend without the guilt of frosting-in-a-jar Nutella. Just make sure the bread, toast, waffle, breakfast cookie, or pancake is gluten-free.

Leftovers for breakfast?

There is nothing wrong with eating last night's leftover salmon fritter or any other meat.

Round out your plate with fresh, wilted greens or last night's green beans. It's all good! Just make sure your plate reflects the basic template.

Smoothie breakfast?

Smoothie recipes are almost as numerous as the stars in the sky, but smoothies can sometimes be nothing more than a glorified hit of sweet carbs in the form of fruit. But a smoothie can *easily* reflect the proportions of The Perfect Plate. Check out the Starter Recipe section for a few ideas.

The Perfect Plate Lunch

Lunch at work?

I spent years watching co-workers with the normal array of modern ailments and diseases repeatedly rely on pre-fabricated nukable "meals." For special occasions, they would gather a group order for a fast-food chain and one worker would come back with a stash of hamburgers, fries, and soft drinks. And don't forget the chips. Nothing in that meal to boost their energy or improve their health.

Dare to be different. Only *you* are at the helm of your health and the *only one* who feels the results of your choices; but remember also to consider your family. They feel your dis-ease when you are not at your best with them. We are not an island...

Bring food from your kitchen. Leftovers were my main go-to for eating lunch at work.

Because I am not a fan of microwaving food, most of my lunches were in a cold form. Leftover veggies and meat with homemade salad dressing filled the bill. Outright salads were favorites as well. Just make sure you have plenty of protein and good fats from meat, fish, poultry, eggs, nuts, seeds, and avocado.

The same way my low carb breakfast held me from 6:30 am to noon, a low carb lunch kept me from the zombie march to the snack machine for sweets, salt, or carbs by 3 pm.

Enjoying stable blood sugars is awesome. I used to be well-stocked with peanut butter or cheese nabs all of the time. I was never sure when I would run out of sugar and need to eat something immediately to stop the trembling, the flush, and the inability to concentrate. Little did I know then, my "fix" of nabs or a sugary peanut bar was only going to contribute to another crash later on.

After dropping most sugar, all glutens, and most starchy carbs, I continue to enjoy stable energies and blood sugars all day long. A novel feeling. I can't imagine *volunteering* to lose that feeling even one day! Can you?

Smoothies and wraps for lunch at home or at work:

Nothing could be easier than a smoothie. They are easily made and can be effortlessly transported to work in a mason jar. Make a large batch the night before. Great for meals or snacks anytime. Before drinking, just shake that Mason jar (lid on!), open up, and enjoy.

For something gluten-free yet sandwich-y, try Paleo Wraps. Made with coconut meat, with or without Turmeric (an awesome spice that is anti-inflammatory), these wraps transform meat and veggie hand-held enjoyment. Paleo Wraps really hold up and could even be used to "embrace" your bacon-egg-sausage scramble for breakfast. Check my Resources section on how to get these from Thrive Market.

Heating up a serving of my rich chicken broth, replete with non-starchy "dumplings" and lots of veggies, is a year round lunch favorite. Every few weeks, I just crave a fresh batch of this wholesome goodness for my bones and over-all nutrition. I gave you a couple versions of this healing broth in the Starter Recipe section.

The Perfect Plate Dinner

This is where it gets even easier. Meat? Done! Half a plate of veggies? Done! Avocado? Done! Maybe a small serving of berries? Or a small salad with avocado, berries, and topped with sprouted seeds or nuts and a homemade dressing with healthy oils? Done and done!

If you want a snack a bit later, check out the recipe for trail mix or my latest favorite for chia jam or pudding. Even two tablespoons of chia seeds stirred into 3/4 cup of hot water with a teaspoon of dried fruit makes a satisfying, staying, snack that will go a long way to regular bowel habits. Loaded with Omega 3s, protein, and fiber—who could want more? The chia seeds will thicken the hot water, and the seeds soften as you stir. Easy and fun.

Looking for a starch treat that won't kick blood sugars through the roof? Three ideas here:

1. Pan-fried, sliced plantains. Use flavorful, organic coconut oil to cover the bottom of the pan. Season with "sweet spices" discussed in the next chapter "Foods and Cooking 101." A small serving of plantains can round out a plate of meat and veggies with a different texture and gentle flavor.

2. Follow the instructions in "Foods and Cooking 101" to indulge in some starchy vegetable such as potato or rice; yet avoid the "carb" hit through the wonders of refrigeration. Learn how soon.

3. Sweet potatoes. Very allowable and nutrient dense. Just don't think in terms of Aunt Martha's sweet potato fluff with a cup of brown sugar and a cup or more of marshmallows. Baked sweet potatoes— especially those cute fingerlings—not only make a colorful addition to the plate but can serve as an awesome snack. "Butter" them with a little coconut oil. My grandchildren love them!

Take Away Thoughts:

- You will be amazed how a starch-free breakfast will hold you for hours of energy filled, clear-headed, high performance.

- Remember the 80/20 Rule and don't sweat the small stuff unless you are allergic.

Take Away Actions:

- Start transforming your meals with breakfast. The way you feel will spur you on to transform the rest of your meals.

Keep the Perfect Plate Template firmly in mind when creating your meals. In fact, post the downloadable copy of it from your Bonus Materials on the refrigerator. **GO HERE** (https://booklaunch.io/deidre/toolkit-for-wellness) for your copy.

How about some tips and guidance to ensure your success and ramp-up flavor? In the next section, you will be learning some kitchen secrets to get the most out of your food for maximum flavor and nutrition. I will be revealing some flavor enhancers that have secret benefits. Food is such fun! Let's get going!

FOODS, COOKING, AND CONDIMENTS 101

This section is designed so you can gain a general philosophy and approach to food preparation that will start you off in a solid wellness direction. I am not going to teach a novice how to cook in one chapter. If you are a novice though, you will be able to gain a bit of confidence and a starting point in Cooking 101.

Approach cooking with an open mind. The same way people use negative thinking about artistic involvement saying, "I can't even draw a straight line!" others refrain from using the stove top saying, "I can't even boil water!" Except for making tea, I hardly ever heat up pots of water. In fact, I have a chapter in this book titled, "Never Boil Again"! Cooking is basic, fundamental, and even earthy. If you were not brought up helping and learning in the kitchen, it's not too late to start on your own.

To really get control of your health and wellness, some home cooking is in order. Fast food, prepared "nukables," and "drop this plastic bag into the water," type of cooking, are flat out not good for you. The time you save from convenience "food," is time cut off from your quality and quantity of life.

Here's the brain thing again. Are you going to be a part of the problem or part of the answer? Learning requires a change in behavior. Okay, you are learning certain foods are not good for you; so you are going to learn how to prepare food that *is* good for you? You are always in control.

Congratulations for committing to take positive steps for your entire state of wellness! In this section, you will be learning many "Easy Tweaks" for food that will pave the way to a calming, digestible, anti-inflammatory diet that will do wonders for your physical well-being. When our physical bodies are running smoothly, our mental and spiritual selves rejoice as well.

The following are some things to generally keep in mind during meal planning and preparation that will help tweak you away from the constant steering toward added sugar and starch, and will help maximize the nutrient density of your meals. Each of these contains secrets I am glad to share for your benefit.

The Secret of Sweet Spices

To create an aura of sweetness, I reach for what I call sweet spices: Cinnamon (which helps regulate blood sugar), nutmeg, cardamom, ginger, allspice, pumpkin pie spice, and Chinese Five Spice. Using these will automatically make the taste buds think "sweet." I also use vanilla and almond extracts in many dishes to add to the sweet effect.

In preparing French toast with gluten-free bread, for example, I always put at least cinnamon and vanilla (to taste) into the egg bath mixture. This way, the spice and vanilla extract will make me think of sweet goodness and I will not need to add any syrup when I eat it. Using coconut oil to fry the French toast will also add another layer of satisfaction to the palate.

Consider cinnamon's many talents:

- Mimics sweetness

- Is loaded with antioxidants

- Calms down inflammation

- Is shown to improve key risk factors for heart disease

- Can reduce insulin resistance and help with blood sugar levels

- Has been shown to decrease the amount of glucose that enters the blood stream after eating, and

- Has been linked to maintaining and helping brain cells.

My research suggests the best form of cinnamon has been shown to be the Ceylon, or "true" cinnamon, which is not the type usually found in the grocery store and is of the Cassia variety.

Garlic and Allium Family Secrets

Garlic is particularly beneficial as an anti-inflammatory, whether inflammation is seen in the skin or felt internally. Garlic is also packed with antioxidants which boost our immune system; and it has anti-fungal properties! Even the ancients knew garlic was a super food. Not only is it a great flavor enhancer, but its anti-inflammatory health benefits abound.

Find ways to add fresh garlic in just about anything. It's one of the first ingredients to go into my chicken broth. Adding some minced garlic is a great flavor enhancer to just about any vegetable and is a delight even in scrambled eggs.

Here's the big secret! Garlic, onions, shallots, leeks, chives and other members of the allium family of vegetables need to rest 10-15 minutes after cutting and before heating to allow for the activation of the enzyme allicin. This enzyme helps in the formation of the beneficial anti-inflammatory properties of these super foods. So maximize what you're after—the healing properties of garlic—and prep garlic and the rest of the allium family first before prepping other items to be cooked. They need resting time to activate that good enzyme. Who knew? Now YOU do! You're welcome!

Ginger Secrets

Ginger is a great thing to add to your anti-inflammatory arsenal. Feeling like the sniffles are coming? Brew fresh ginger, green tea, lemon juice, and a touch of honey for a tea that will go a long way to smoothing unhappy sinuses and throats! Ginger can actually inhibit the common cold virus, rhinovirus. Prepare for the cold and flu season by sipping on this tea regularly. Take your flu shot, too.

Another big benefit of this fabulous root is as an anti-inflammatory, it can be an upset tummy's best friend. It calms nausea, improves digestion in general, and even helps stimulate appetite! That's why ginger is the second added ingredient in the Quick Healing Chicken Soup recipe.

Turmeric Secrets

Turmeric, also known as curcumin, is an ancient healing ingredient with amazing anti-inflammatory properties similar to ginger. According to Dr. Andrew Weil who summarized James A. Duke's highly respected studies on turmeric, there are at least three main diseases that this root combats:

1. Alzheimer's disease: Turmeric actually helps to block the very formation of the beta-amyloid plaques from forming in the brain which hallmark the Alzheimer's brain deterioration process.

2. Arthritis: Studies show substantial relief of the symptoms of arthritis through the anti-inflammatory action of turmeric.

3. Cancer: Duke University, one of the nation's leading health facilities, pointed to over two hundred scientific citations for benefits of turmeric with cancer and seven hundred citations for curcumin and cancer.

If regular consumption of turmeric in curry dishes is not enough, turmeric supplements are available. Dr. Weil suggests 400-600 mg of extracts three times a day or as the label may indicate. Always work with your doctor or nutritionist when adding supplements.

Chia Seed Secrets

Chia seeds. Possibly the 8th wonder of the world!

Consider this nutritional profile for 2 tablespoons of chia seeds:

- Protein keeps you full and decreases appetite, two times the protein of other grains or seeds.

- Calcium, calming and beneficial to bones, 5 times the calcium of milk with 18% of the RDA

- Omega-3 fatty acids, very anti-inflammatory and beneficial, 5 grams

- Fiber, essential for smooth functioning bowels, 11 grams; 40% fiber by weight

- Net carbohydrates, which we do not want in abundance, 1 gram

- 30% RDA of manganese, magnesium, and 27% RDA of phosphorus

- Full of anti-oxidants

- Slow absorption which keeps you feeling full and satisfied.

The Secret of Resistant Starch

By now, you may be thinking starch is something to be avoided in any great quantities because of the whole high blood sugar and insulin thing. You're right! But resistant starch is being called a third kind of fiber. It goes through the small intestine unchanged and unabsorbed. Resistant starch then goes to the colon where it feeds the "good" bacteria.

In your *Toolkit for Wellness,* I am emphasizing maintaining an anti-inflammatory diet to maintain the integrity of the lining of the small intestine. The other benefit of this way of eating is the enormous benefit of maintaining a healthy environment for good gut bacteria to flourish. Writing about our gut environment, its "microbiome," is a book for another day. But, rest assured, an anti-inflammatory diet is the keystone to a happy microbiome.

So, resistant starch (RS) can be best learned about in MarksDailyApple.com where Mark Sisson will give you the whole technical scoop about it. He will describe how RS increases insulin sensitivity, decreases fasting blood sugars, increases absorption for magnesium, and decreases leaky gut.

The bottom line for our purposes and the secret: You can tap into the benefits of RS by eating rice or potatoes that have *first* been cooked *and* cooled before consumption. Hello potato salad made with real ingredient mayonnaise! See resources section for connecting with Thrive Market for Primal Mayo.

Secrets for an Asian Flair without Soy Sauce

An anti-inflammatory diet can still boast all of the good taste that comes with Asian dishes without using soy sauce which contains gluten from wheat. Wheat-free Tamari, along with coconut aminos, confer the qualities of soy sauce without the wheat pollution.

Also look for gluten-free fish sauce which adds that fifth taste called "umami." I have learned to add a teaspoon or so of fish sauce to my tomato-based sauces to impart that yummy goodness factor. No fish taste. I use Red Boat Fish Sauce available through Thrive Market (see resources section).

Also try finishing steamed vegetables—especially broccoli—with a small amount of dark toasted sesame oil! Hmm!

Secrets for Thickening Sauces

Arrowroot is my go-to thickening agent. It totally replaces corn starch. Whether it is turkey giblet gravy (see Special Times chapter) or thickening to my Asian Stir Fry (see Recipes), just stir arrowroot into a bit of water and add to your sauce while stirring. No corn.

Secrets of Open-Faced, Gluten-Free Sandwiches

Yes, Virginia, there are gluten-free sandwiches! Choosing to not include gluten in your diet is no reason to feel totally bread deprived. In addition to abundant resources and recipes for home baking, there are—usually frozen—breads and rolls available that are tasty and gluten-free.

The nature and texture of these breads without the "glue" from gluten changes the two slice sandwich dynamic for me. I am just as satisfied with a single slice, open-faced sandwich; otherwise, it's just too bread-y, which is really a good thing because starch is starch, gluten-free or not.

Fresh homemade gluten-free breads are delicious for sandwiches. If it's fresh and warm from the oven, gluten-free bread is great. The next day, the bread needs to be either toasted or pan grilled—my favorite—for it to be at its best. In other words, packing most kinds of gluten-free bread for a meal later in the day is just not the same if it can't be warmed somehow.

The exception to this is Danielle Walker's recipe for World Famous Sandwich Bread in her *Against All Grain* cookbook. Her secret ingredient is cashew butter. This bread stays moist. It can be sliced very thin for a return to two-slice sandwiches. It still bends and holds together even with super-thin slices.

Take Away Thoughts:

- If you are an old hand at cooking, you may be discovering new ways to direct your skills that will definitely enhance the nutrient density of the foods you eat and serve. There is something other than bread and wheat everything. There are other ways to flavor food without sugar.

- There are so many people of every age who are new to food prep and cooking at home. The positive results from eating ingredients that are "real," not packaged, shrink-wrapped, or instantly "cooked" in a microwave, will spur you on because of the amazing way you will feel. Divesting yourself from the onslaught of chemicals, dyes, wheat, and sugar will transform you.

Take Away Actions:

- Explore the wonders of "sweet spices" and flavorings to enjoy French toast and pancakes without syrup.

- Add that umami factor to just about everything using a teaspoon of gluten-free fish sauce. Truly a secret ingredient that will ramp up flavor in magical ways.

- Extract all of the benefits of garlic and others in the allium family by cutting, grating, and prepping at least 10-15 minutes before heating.

Armed with all of these "secrets," we can move on to tips about putting these ingredients together in the easiest way possible and how to store them to ensure their safe quality.

Some Assembly Required

Well, you have opened up your Wellness Kit, become familiar with all of the tools and how to use them, and now you come across some instructions bearing those words that all parents dread on Christmas Eve night: Some assembly required. Yes, folks, if you want that pretty red tricycle under the tree by morning, somebody is going to need to put things together!

Not to worry, dear readers. You can put food on the table and in your bellies that does not come from a box, a nukable tray, or an easy-boil pouch. Fear not! You have some easy-to-follow cooking basics that will do you well. Cooking from scratch does not have to require slaving in the kitchen for hours on end, nor does it require extensive culinary skills.

Here are some ideas to help you get started in the world of self-prepared food if you are a "newbie." If you are an old hand at cooking, please read the part below about plastics that will give you an idea about supporting your good health.

My most used pans are small, medium, and large-sized enameled sauté pans. A little good fat or oil, some veggies, some meat, medium heat, and you're done. The work comes in cutting up veggies and keeping the workspace neat. There's a soup pot, too, of course; but when I look at what is used most in my vast array of equipment, it's not that much. Cooking is not astrophysics. A food processor helps, as does a high speed blender (Vitamix).

Cooking pans are either stainless steel or cast iron. Aluminum pans just scare me regarding the transfer of aluminum and linkages to Alzheimer's disease. Sauté pans should be coated in something other than Teflon which can release hazardous fumes with higher heat. It is getting a lot easier to find pans coated with an enamel finish for a non-stick effect.

Storing food in glass containers is preferable to plastic because of the toxins in plastic. Some of those toxins have been identified as butylated hydroxyanisole, (BHA); but the replacements for those toxins have not been evaluated over the long term. Cooking in plastic is out, too, because the transfer of toxins is enhanced with the heating of plastic containers.

We are seeing more and more problems with hormone imbalances; and I have read there is a link with our penchant for using plastics with our food and hormone dysregulation. I remember the days when we saved every plastic container imaginable to store food in. Then we got smart and bought nicer looking plastic containers so everything matched. With the advent of the microwave, we were quick to check if our plastic containers were "nukable." Enter an uptick in all sorts of diseases research is now linking to plastic.

I have finally booted out the last of the plastic storage containers by buying a great assortment of glass containers with four-sided snap down locking lids at Costco. I will soon be returning to get yet another set or two for storing my grain-free flours and nuts. It's all a process, one step at a time in the right direction. A glass storage system would make a wonderful gift, especially to those just starting out so they can protect their health right from the start. Certainly, it's never too late to convert.

A set of different-sized cutting boards, a set of knives, wooden spoons, bowl scraping spatulas, and a pancake turner and you are set to go. Other equipment can come with time and need. See? You can do this!

If daily food preparation is not your speed, cooking in large batches is tremendously beneficial to working people. The results of weekend cooking sprees can be enjoyed all week long or longer if the freezer is used along with those glass containers with snap on lids! I love preparing "vats" of soups, sauces, and gravies and parceling them out in meal sizes for future use from the freezer. Leftovers have become my best friend! They easily convert to breakfast side-dishes. They become the foundation for workday lunches and salads. They are great as a starting point for the next dinner time.

Involving the whole family is tops in my book for bonding, sharing, team work, appreciating the culinary efforts it takes to create a meal, and in expanding the family spirit of exploration. This is how skills of self-reliance are born. To put a spin on an old adage, "Give a child a meal and you feed him once. Show a child how to prepare healthful foods and he will feed himself for a very long, healthy lifetime!"

With your "can do!" attitude, let's explore how to guarantee your success at fueling your body and your whole family with the best possible nutritional energy. You are going to create your "Environment for Success." It's a concept that works with food; and its principles can be applied to any area of your life in which you are striving for successful changes. Read on!

Take Away Thoughts:

- Even the equipment we use can contribute to our wellness or state of dis-ease. The surge of so many auto-immune diseases has been in lock-step with our use of aluminum and plastic. You can make better choices for your health and the health of your whole family.

Take Away Actions:

- Switch to glass whenever possible.

- Do not cook in plastic.

- Throw out that plastic!

- Convert to enamel coatings for pans.

The next section of this chapter will 'seal the deal' for your success. Without a doubt, this next step is the keystone to making your new food habits easy to incorporate into your daily life. Relying on willpower will be a thing of the past. Hello, success!

An Environment for Success!

Wouldn't it be great if you could gain an advantage that would make your dietary habit changes a lot easier without having to shore up your resolve? Here comes a key thing to do which will eliminate tempting distractions. I remember doing this and it was so liberating! Doing this gave me a firm sense of control and POWER!

Okay. If success in eating for wellness is your goal, let's make sure you will succeed. If, for instance, you did not want to eat candy, working in a Godiva chocolate shop would be a very difficult environment for success at your goal. If you wanted to quit smoking, stepping outside at work with smokers on break might make you want to join in again.

Choosing to make positive choices for your health and happiness is important. Your kitchen cupboards should reflect your new values. Your kitchen should *not* look like what's on the shelves of a Seven-Eleven convenience store.

Do not wait until you have "eaten all of the bad stuff up." That will never happen and you'll just buy more. Didn't you make a commitment to your body to look out for it? To listen to it? To "have its back"? So prove it!

I promised the positive changes outlined in this book would not require sheer willpower. Relying on willpower itself is pretty much a sure fire recipe for failure over the long run. Making positive changes for your wellness should stoke you to do *more*, not whisper in your ear you are a failure when you get tempted.

What has caused past disappointments can be circumvented by following my tips about tweaking habits, mindful breathing, stress reduction strategies, creating a positive connection with your wellness, employing positive brain power, simple and doable exercise, mindful food choices based on your new understanding about how nutrients work in your body, AND in creating an environment for success!

To prevent those times when you have to employ sheer willpower not to reach for the chips or cookies, you simply have to get rid of them. Unopened containers can go to a food drive; opened items can either just be thrown away, or fed to the birds and squirrels. I remember going through my cupboards. It was also a chance to get rid of things that were way out of date. It turned out my emergency stock pile was mostly toxic and old. In a best case scenario, your whole family can join in the fun. Purging the shelves, cupboards, refrigerator, and automobile stashes of junk snack food is the great first step on your journey in improved health.

Having an accountability partner is also a recipe for success. In addition to your family, enlisting a friend to join you in reclaiming health can give a real boost to your progress through mutual accountability, encouragement, praise, and sharing creativity. You can make small habit tweaks together, walk together, share recipes, and success.

Of course, I am here for you, too. My contact information is at the end of this book. Helping you is why I am writing this in the first place. Hearing of your successes, challenges, questions, and your own tips is what makes this all worthwhile. I want to help you on your journey to fulfill your dream of feeling better in every way.

Take Away Thoughts:

- We tell our children to make friends with a better crowd because we know whoever they are around will influence them, and bad tends to drag down good. We cannot expect ourselves to improve what we are feeding our bodies if we are surrounded by chips, sodas, and donuts. Success is yours if you "dress" your kitchen and cupboards for success.

Take Away Actions:

- Make it easy on yourself by creating an environment for success. It's easier to reach for a handful of activated nuts for a snack—which you will hardly ever need because you are satisfied until the next meal—if nuts or sanely constructed trail mix is the only choice to make.

- Be social about this. Do not keep this great news to yourself. Helping another person is such a blessing and your partnership will help you both with accountability, support, and ideas. Share your *Toolkit for Wellness* with a friend and take the journey together!

You are off the hook if "you can't even boil water". Learn why, next, and hold your head up high!

Never Boil Again!

You know the expression, "They can't even boil water"? Well, that's great, because boiling water is not needed or desired!

Have you ever been to a fair or home expo where there are cooking demonstrations? We went to one where a certain brand of pots and pans was being extolled. They are great pans. I've been happily using mine for thirty years.

The demonstration was memorable for me when they compared side-by-side taste tests of carrots they had cooked in front of our eyes. In one pan, they boiled the carrots the way we all probably grew up seeing and doing. In the other pan, they actually used no water at all and cooked the carrots slowly using their own moisture.

All of us watching were able to taste the results of each method. Blah carrots versus carrots that were singing with flavor!

I never boiled carrots or any other vegetable again. Vegetables have become stand-outs for flavor at our house. A purchase of waterless cooking pans is not necessarily required. This nutrition and flavor saving method can be done with standard pans with just a couple tablespoons of water to barely cover the bottom and using a medium low heat. Or, just gently sauté vegetables in a healthy oil, followed by putting a lid on the pan for a steam finish.

Not only is using a minimum of water going to result in great tasting veggies, but the nutrients we are after will be staying in the vegetables and not leaving in the cooking water. Another win-win! The more we can enjoy fantastic flavor, the more we will want to eat nutrient dense vegetables.

Take Away Thought:

- We are eating to get nutrients, right?

Take Away Action:

- Stop boiling!

STARTER RECIPES

Smoothies

Smoothie Choices

Smoothies can be a convenient way to pack in the nutrients in something easy to prepare, easy to transport, and easy to ingest. They can also be a wolf in sheep's clothing; they are about nutrition, not added sugar. If you add a protein powder to your smoothie, make sure it's not loaded with carbohydrates. For serious weight loss, it has been recommended to stick with 50 grams of carbohydrates a day, not per meal.

You can get a good serving of fruit, green veggies, fiber, protein, good fats, and all the vitamins, minerals, and tons of anti-this and pro-that all in one glass.

A good, heavy-duty blender like a Vitamix will take your smoothies to the next level! They are a worthy investment, and you can get totally reliable remanufactured ones. No more grainy smoothies.

Basic Smoothie Ingredient Choices

Fruit: All kinds of berries rule, including kiwi! Some banana is good and cherries, too. Slow down on excess banana, pineapple, papaya and the like because of their high glycemic index.

Fat: can be in the form of a nut butter, nuts, coconut milk/cream, coconut flakes, avocado, or seeds

Protein: can come from the nuts and seeds (don't forget flax, chia, and hemp) but also as powdered additive (see caution above about carb count)

Veggies: Try to switch these around a bit so as not to have kale each day—spinach, kale, or salad greens; some people go for beets or carrots, even!

Flavorings: A pinch of salt wouldn't be amiss, as well as some "sweet spices" (cinnamon, nutmeg, cardamom, Chinese 5 Spice). Vanilla or almond extract is always a plus.

Fluid: water, coconut water, coconut milk, and almond milk

Extras: fresh mint leaves, yogurt, canned pumpkin puree, cucumber, fresh ginger, cocoa powder, and unflavored gelatin

*A note about nuts and seeds: soak what raw nuts and larger seeds you will be using for several hours before use to activate the enzymes that ease and maximize digestion.

The Thrive Market Smoothie

1 cup coconut water

1/2 cup or more baby spinach

1 frozen banana, I use just 1/2 banana

1 cup frozen blueberries

1 Medjool date, pitted

2 tablespoons hemp seeds

1 tablespoon chia seeds

Place all ingredients together in blender and blend on high until well mixed. Serve and enjoy!

Flavored Water

Especially if you are new to drinking water—yes, those people exist—you may want something more from your water other than the pure joy of great hydration. You can acquire a taste for water; but if you need a boost, here are a few ideas other than Southern (say SWEET) iced tea.

Before going to bed, put your flavor ingredients into a glass container, fill with water, put in refrigerator, and get ready to enjoy in the morning.

Make sure the fruits and herbs are very clean of bugs and/or toxins. Organic items would be safer by far. Muddle leaves by using the back of a spoon to smash/rub the leaves on the side of the container. Fruits can be slightly muddled to release some of their juices.

Mint leaves: Make sure to muddle the leaves before adding water to release the flavor-containing oils

Cucumber, mint leaves, lime: Slice up 2-3 inches of cucumber, muddle a few mint leaves, slice some lime

Strawberries, lemon, basil: Slice several berries, ½ lemon and ¼ cup basil leaves (muddle everything)

Lemon: Use the juice of ½ of a lemon and slice up the rest

Ginger: Slice about 1 inch piece of fresh ginger and smash slices like garlic cloves before putting into container

Raspberry, lime: Gather up a handful of raspberries, along with at least one lime. Squeeze juice into container and then add the squeezed quarters.

Pineapple, mint: Simply add about ½ cup fresh, cubed pineapple to the muddled mint

Blackberry, sage: A handful of blackberries added to desired amount of fresh muddled sage is good

Orange, mint: Slice a whole or half of an orange and use desired amount of muddled mint

Watermelon: Drop a few chunks of ice cold watermelon into a glass to create, not only a delicious beverage, but a festive one as well!

Breakfast

Breakfast Cookies

Adapted from a recipe by Danielle Walker

This is a large recipe that makes about 27 cookies using two large parchment covered cookie sheets. I use an 11-cup food processor to mix most of this, followed by a final stirring using a large bowl to incorporate the two batches of ingredients. The **bold face** alternate ingredients make this recipe into **Pumpkin Spice Breakfast Cookies**.

In a food processor, place the following ingredients and pulse 2-3 times for 15 seconds each pulse until dates are in very small pieces and bananas are smooth:

1 Tbsp. Lemon juice

3 large, ripe bananas broken into chunks

7 medium-sized dates /or/ 5 large Medjool dates, soaked in warm water for 15 minutes and drained

2 Tbsp. ghee /or/ palm shortening

1 cup unsweetened applesauce OR **pumpkin puree**

Pour the majority of this mixture into a large bowl; scraping is not needed. Then place the following ingredients into the processor bowl and pulse for 5-6 bursts until incorporated:

1 cup of hazelnut /or/ almond flour* OR **2/3 cup almond and 1/3 cup coconut flour**

1/4 cup ground flax seed

1/4 cup hemp seed hearts

1/4 cup Great Lakes gelatin, Collagen Hydrolysate (does not cause gelling)

3 tsp. cinnamon

2 tsp. vanilla extract

2 tsp. baking soda

Add the following to the nut flour mixture and pulse 3-4 bursts until incorporated:

1 cup unsweetened coconut flakes

1/2 cup dried fruit of choice—usually berries OR **golden raisins**

Add contents of food processor to those in the large bowl and hand mix using a large wooden spoon or spatula until well-combined. The batter is a bit wet, but should hold its shape well. If it seems too wet, add some coconut flour 1 tablespoonful at a time.

Using a golf ball-sized cookie scoop, scoop out and place cookies onto parchment paper covered cookie sheets.

Using damp fingers, gently press each one down a bit.

Bake at 350 degrees for 20-25 minutes. I use a convection oven, which automatically lowers the temp to 325 degrees. A regular oven may change the timing. Cookies will still be a little bit soft but not mushy when done. Place cookies on a cooling rack where they will firm up.

A couple of these make an awesome breakfast, especially when spread with almond butter alone or almond butter mixed with a tad of Justin's Chocolate Hazelnut Butter. Justin's version of Nutella has organic cane sugar as the *third* ingredient after hazelnuts and almonds and contains only 8 grams of sugar compared to the other's 21 grams of sugar as the *first* ingredient!

* I have used various combinations of flours depending upon what I had in stock. Coconut flour will dry dough, so the amount of moistness will change depending on how much coconut flour you use. If the dough is wet, add a spoonful of coconut flour at a time as you stir it in to the batter.

Morning Glory Power Muffins

Yield: 20 muffins

Preheat oven to 350 degrees

Ingredients

1/2 cup golden raisins

4 Tbsp. hemp seed hearts

3 Tbsp. ground golden flax seed meal

3/4 cup unsweetened coconut flakes

1 cup grated carrots

1 cup crushed pineapple no sugar added

1 cup chopped walnuts*

2 medium-sized ripe bananas, mashed

1/3 cup brown sugar

1-1/2 tsp. vanilla

3 eggs

1 tsp. cinnamon

1/4 tsp. ground ginger ¼ tsp. kosher salt

1-1/2 tsp. baking soda

1 cup gluten-free flour

1/2 tsp. xanthan gum

1/4 cup coconut flour

1/3 cup coconut oil, melted

*always use activated nuts—see recipe

Method

In a large mixing bowl and using an electric mixer, beat the eggs until creamy yellow; add the banana, vanilla, brown sugar, cinnamon, ginger, salt, and baking soda, beating until well combined. Add the melted coconut oil and mix well. Beat in the flours and xanthan gum.

Then, using a wooden spoon or spatula, stir in the raisins, hemp, flax seed, coconut, carrot, pineapple, and walnuts. Make sure to mix all ingredients well.

Fill baking cup lined muffin tins about 3/4 full.

Bake in pre-heated, 350 degree oven for 28 minutes or until a toothpick comes out clean after being inserted.

I hope you agree these are the "best ever Morning Glories"! Their power comes from the hemp, flax, and walnuts which give great forms of "good fat" as in Omega 3 fatty acids and protein. Certainly, the other ingredients aren't too shabby, either!

Quick Paleo Pancakes

1 Banana

2 Eggs

Salt, to taste

Cinnamon, to taste

Vanilla extract, to taste

This can be stirred up in a blender, a food processor, or just smashed up with a fork and blended! Pour into a hot pan greased with a healthy oil and you have pancakes that are already sweet and savory. Only addition might be some Justin's Brand Chocolate Hazelnut Butter on top!

Veggies

Brussels Sprouts with Cranberries and Prosciutto or Bacon

Ingredients

1 Bag Brussels sprouts, washed, stem and outer leaves removed, sliced or cut into quarters

2-3 slices of prosciutto torn into small pieces /or/ 2-3 slices of bacon cooked and crumbled

1-2 Tbsp. ghee (used in the pan)

¼ cup dried cranberries

¼ medium onion, sliced and diced—optional

Sea salt, to taste

1-2 Tbsp. water

Optional: 1-2 Tbsp. balsamic vinegar

Method

Heat ghee in large sauté pan and add prepared Brussels sprouts (and onion, if using).

Stir occasionally until the sprouts become bright green. Add salt, cranberries, and 1-2 Tbsp. water; put lid on pan and reduce heat a bit to allow steaming process. When cooked to the desired doneness, stir in the prosciutto or bacon, and serve.

If desired, when the sprout mixture is done cooking, remove lid, raise heat a bit, and add the balsamic vinegar. Stir occasionally, letting the moisture reduce. Add the prosciutto or bacon, and serve.

Sesame, Leek, Onion, and Bok Choy Stir Fry

Ingredients

1 Leek

1/4 large onion

1 Bundle of baby Bok choy with three bunches

1/2 inch fresh ginger, peeled and finely minced

2 Cloves garlic, minced

2 Tbsp. extra virgin olive oil

2 Tbsp. toasted sesame oil

1-2 tsp. sesame seeds

Method

Prepare the leek by slicing it in half lengthwise and holding each half under running water, fanning the leaves to remove any grit.

Slice the leeks across the grain, resulting in little half rounds.

Slice the ¼ large onion to give a similar shape as the leek slices.

Carefully wash the baby Bok choy and slice across to give a similar shape to the other veggies.

Put olive oil in large sauté pan, add onions and leeks, cooking over medium heat. Stir occasionally until the onions start to become translucent.

Add the Bok choy and continue stirring occasionally. As the Bok choy starts to wilt and become brilliant dark green, add the toasted sesame oil, minced garlic, and the minced ginger.

When all of the ingredients have been combined and are fragrant, serve and garnish with sesame seeds.

Carrot, Beet, Parsnip Fritters

This is a great time to pull out the food processor with the grater attachment! Just keep feeding in the veggies and dump the grated results a few times into a large mixing bowl.

The rest is just toss, squeeze, and pan fry!

Ingredients

2 carrots, peeled and grated

1 parsnip, peeled and grated

1 beet, peeled and grated

1/4 of a large onion, grated

1-2 eggs

1-2 large cooking/serving spoons full of coconut flour

Salt and pepper to taste

Olive oil to coat the bottom of skillet

Method

Toss the grated veggies well to combine. Add first egg and first large spoonful of coconut flour along with seasonings. Mix well to incorporate all ingredients. I just used my gloved hands throughout this process. If your mixture looks like it needs more "glue" to stick together into patties, add the additional egg and coconut flour. Quantities vary depending upon the size of the veggies.

I then form the patties. Using a hamburger press might be a good idea to try. Just beware there will be beautiful, drippy, red juice coming out of the patties as you squeeze, which is best do over another bowl or the sink.

Place patties in a hot skillet with olive oil and fry a few minutes on each side.

If your beet came with its leafy top, wash, chop, and sauté the tops in olive oil and season with sea salt, and a bit of crushed red pepper! Yum!

Savory Parsnip Fries

Peel and cut about 4 parsnips into 3-4 inch fry shapes and place in bowl

Melt 2 Tbsp. of ghee and pour over fries

Sprinkle ½ Tbsp. of curry powder, salt and pepper to taste over fries

Toss or mix the fries to coat evenly

Place fries in a single layer on parchment lined baking sheet

Bake in oven set at 350 degrees for about 15 minutes. Stir fries around. Continue baking for about 15 minutes more until golden and crispy.

Spicy Carrot Fries

Peel and cut about 5-6 carrots into 3-4 inch fry shapes and place in bowl

Drizzle approximately 2 Tbsp. olive oil over fries so that they are evenly coated after stirring them around

Sprinkle the following seasonings over the fries in amounts to taste:

Paprika, cayenne pepper, garlic powder, chili powder, salt, and pepper

Stir seasoned fries to coat all sides with seasonings

Place fries in a single layer on parchment-lined baking sheet

Bake in oven set at 350 degrees for about 15 minutes. Stir fries around. Continue baking for about 15 minutes more until crispy.

Zoodles

Zoodles are not a recipe, but things! Zoodles are one of the best alternatives to starchy pasta, can be used cooked or raw, are super-fun to make, especially if you have a spiralizer; and will make using up those prolific zucchini and other summer squash a breeze! They are an easy way to add veggies to any dinner plate or summer buffet.

Here are some zoodles tips:

- You can pre-peel the squash or not

- Create zoodles with a julienne peeler or spiral slicer

- Place zoodles in a colander and toss with about 1 tsp of sea salt and allow to rest for up to ½ hour. This coaxes the extra moisture out of the zoodles so your plate won't be soupy.

- Squeeze the zoodles dry. Paper towels work, but I prefer using a clean kitchen towel or bath towel to spread out the zoodles, roll up, and gently squeeze. The drier, the better.

The rest is up to you! Here are some zoodles ideas:

- Don't boil! Just lightly sauté

- Use as a replacement for spaghetti noodles. Lightly sauté in olive oil until al dente

- Use sweet basil pesto while cooking for a stand-alone veggie

- Or combine with shrimp also cooked in sweet basil pesto for a fabulous entrée

- Cook with minced garlic or garlic powder

- Experiment with different seasoning combinations, perhaps Penzey's Bavarian

- Spice with a splash of toasted sesame oil to finish

- Eat raw as a fun salad with different dressings and additions

Zucchini and Turmeric Fritters

This will not only help you enjoy the bountiful zucchini in the summertime, but will help ramp up anti-inflammatory benefits with the turmeric. Additionally, protein and omega3 fatty acids are the benefits of the hemp seed hearts!

Grate 2 zucchini into a bowl; toss with 1 tsp. salt; let rest for 15-20 minutes; and squeeze dry using a towel. Return zucchini to bowl.

Add 1 large egg along with:

> 1/4 cup hemp seed hearts
>
> 1 teaspoon turmeric
>
> Kosher /or/ sea salt, to taste
>
> Pepper, to taste
>
> 1/3 cup coconut flour

Stir ingredients until well combined. If mixture is too wet, add a bit more coconut flour.

Heat enough coconut or avocado oil to coat bottom of fry pan on medium heat.

Using a large cookie scoop, gather mixture into a ball and drop into fry pan.

Flatten each scoop out just a bit and fry a few minutes on each side until crispy.

Veggie Tips

All you have to do with **fresh asparagus** is roll the stems around in a pan with some pastured butter and salt! They turn a vibrant green and are cooked in minutes! I remember reading Miss Manners saying asparagus spears are a finger food! How fun is that for the kids!

Broccoli is especially good steamed—with or without—a steaming basket. More often than not, I will take a sauce pan, just barely cover the bottom with water, and place a broccoli head, with stem end down, into it. The pan is full of broccoli and the stem is trimmed down so the lid will go on. A bit of Kosher, or sea salt, and you're good to go to slowly steam the broccoli on heat, a bit lower than medium. This vegetable will turn a bright green, and is done when a fork can pierce the stems easily. To finish the broccoli, drizzle a little toasted sesame seed oil on top or butter it with pastured butter. Divine!

Broccoli Rabi is one vegetable for which I make an exception. An intriguing vegetable with a slight, but not offensive, bitterness, they are best quickly blanched in small batches, drained, and then finished by stir frying in avocado oil with garlic! These, too, are best if finished with a drizzle of toasted sesame oil.

Brussels sprouts no longer have to be disguised in melted "cheese products" to cover up their flavor! Get rid of the faux food additives and discover some great flavor! Try frying some nitrate-free bacon first, saving some of the bacon fat in the pan. Sauté sliced or quartered Brussels sprouts in the fat along with a quarter of a chopped onion, salt to taste, and add a clove or two of minced garlic. When the Brussels sprouts and onions are getting tender, add a small handful of dried cranberries and the bacon crumbles. Put a lid on the pan and let steam for a few minutes. This creates a savory and slightly sweet dish that will please!

Green beans will turn bright and flavorful when just sautéed on less than medium heat in a bit of ghee, olive oil, pastured butter, coconut oil, or avocado oil, with pink Himalayan salt; and then lightly steamed at the end by putting the lid on the pan.

Fried okra is a southern staple, but it is always breaded (gluten); and well... it's deep fat fried! I now enjoy all the wonders and benefits of high fiber okra by simply sautéing sliced okra into a pan with good oil. Season with Montreal Seasoning for an awesome treat! I could eat this every day! Just shake the pan every minute or two to brown the okra 'jewels' on all sides!

Soups

Better Bone Broth and Soup

Many people advocate drinking one cup of bone broth everyday as an elixir for everything from stronger bones to improved overall health! Make sure your bone broth is up to snuff and you know how to tell the difference! Using a large stock pot, add the following:

Ingredients for flavoring the broth:

LOTS of bony pieces of meat, preferably from grass fed animals or free range chickens. We're talking more than one rotisserie chicken carcass! Today, I used a family packsized tray of chicken wing parts containing just the two-boned half of the wing, not the single-boned mini drumettes. If possible, add 3-4 chicken feet (just don't tell your family!) which will give added nutrients and the desired "gelling" goodness. For a beef broth, beef knuckles and ox-tails work great. 2-3 carrots cut up into 1-2 inch chunks

2-3 ribs celery cut up into 1-2 inch chunks

1/2 to 1 onion cut up into 1 inch 'square' chunks

2-4 Tbsp. apple cider vinegar which helps extract minerals from the bones

2 Tbsp. unflavored gelatin (I use Great Lakes brand for its purity)

Large handful of fresh parsley, chopped

Salt and pepper to taste

1 tsp. ground porcini mushroom powder for an amazing "umami" factor!

2 tsp. poultry seasoning if using chicken

1-2 bay leaves, fresh thyme and/or oregano, and garlic if using beef 12-24 hours of cooking time, preferably divided.

Method (for Broth)

Fill the remainder of the stock pot with water. I cook my bone broth for about 8 hours one day, cool it off in a cold water bath, refrigerate overnight, skim off congealed fat, check for gelling which shows how far along the way the broth is—the more gelled, the better—and return to a gentle simmer. IF using meaty bones and you want that meat as a part of a _soup_, remove the meat after 2-3 hours of simmering and return the bones, cartilage, and skin to the broth for the rest of the cooking time. Refrigerate the meat and use for the soup making later on. Add the parsley in the last hour or two of the cooking time.

Strain the broth using a large colander to remove big chunks. If desiring a really clear broth for daily drinking, strain again using a fine mesh strainer.

Method (for Soup)

Add fresh cut up vegetables to the strained broth, simmer to desired tenderness, return meat to the soup, adjust seasoning and serve.

Nut Dumplings for Chicken Soup

Now that you have a rich and healthful chicken broth from the preceding recipe, you can create a hearty meal with the addition of nutritionally-dense veggie choices. Add some fun dumplings that will increase the nutritive factor and thicken the soup as well.

Ingredients for Dumplings

1/2 cup tapioca flour

1-1/2 cups slivered /or/ sliced almonds

1/2 tsp. salt

1/2 tsp. poultry seasoning

1/3 cup cooled broth

Method for Dumplings

Using a food processor, grind the almonds into a fine flour. Add the tapioca flour, salt, and poultry seasoning and pulse several times to combine. Add the cooled soup broth and pulse until a soft dough forms. Drop teaspoon-sized dumplings into soup that is at a gentle boil. Cook for about 10 minutes.

Soup Ideas

While bags of frozen veggies are a quick way to 'flesh out' a good soup, chopping up fresh veggies is too! But even if you use a bag of frozen veggies, you definitely will want to add some leafy greens and other sources of great nutrition. Consider these:

- Tear up several sheets of sea weed "paper"
- Add broccoli florets
- Slice up kale, chard, or spinach leaves into strips
- Grate a fresh beet to change the soup to Borscht!
- Add zoodles!
- Add a handful of chopped parsley

Pinched for Time Healthy and Healing Chicken Soup

If you do not have the time for an all-day bone simmering event, then I have discovered a great way that can speed things up yet retain nutrition.

To a large stock pot on medium heat add:

2 cloves garlic, minced or pressed

1 to 1-1/2 inches fresh ginger, grated

1 Tbsp. organic apple cider vinegar

2 Tbsp. Great Lakes gelatin completely dissolved in 1/4 cup boiling water

3-4 pairs of chicken drumsticks with thighs attached

1- 32 oz. container of organic, gluten-free, free-range chicken broth

Enough water to finish covering the chicken, about 3 cups

Cover and bring to a gently boil; lower heat to an active simmer.

When the meat is completely cooked (in about 2 hours), remove from the bones; reserve bones. Chop up cooked chicken. Soup could be ready to serve at this point if you are looking for something healing and easy on the tummy, with or without the meat. Vegetables can be added at this point as well. Whatever broth is left, return bones and cool broth. Put into the refrigerator. When reheating, the bones will add additional goodness as the gelatinous broth is warmed.

Desserts

Magic Mousse

Ingredients for the Magic Mousse

4 oz. dark chocolate

3 oz. water /or/ 2 oz. water and 1 oz. spirits

Pinch of salt

Ingredients for the Magic Whipped Topping

Coconut cream from one can full fat coconut milk that has been chilled 2-3 hours

Vanilla /or/ almond extract

1/2 tsp. sugar—optional

Method

On low heat, slowly melt the chocolate and heat the fluid, stirring to incorporate. Remove from heat. Transfer the melted chocolate mixture into a small bowl and place bowl into an ice bath (ice cubes and water). Using an electric mixer with the whip attachment—beat, beat, beat! This may take 5 minutes, but be patient! All at once the liquid will get thick and then very thick! It will be possible to beat past the mousse point and get something quite firm—in which case, melting and re-whipping will be needed.

Spoon the Magic Mousse into small ramekins (this is very rich and calls for wee tasting spoons).

Once all of the mousse is dished up, use the same bowl with the chocolate mousse scrapings left inside and spoon in the coconut cream from the chilled can of coconut milk. When chilled, it is easy to spoon out the cream. Save the rest for enriching rice, quinoa, or a smoothie! Place the coconut cream bowl into the ice bath and using the same whipping attachment beat, beat, beat! When things start looking like whipped cream, add the vanilla or almond extract and optional sugar and beat some more!

Spoon on or pipe on the topping to finish this amazingly easy dessert! Your guests will be amazed!

Peach Icebox Pie with "Benefits"

This recipe has plenty of bone and joint health benefits of gelatin, and boosts in protein from, not only the gelatin and eggs, but from the flax seed that also gives omega-3 fatty acids! Win! Win! Win!

Prepare the crust first so it can completely cool before adding the contents

Put the following ingredients into a food processor and pulse until well combined:

> 1/2 cup whole flax seeds
>
> 1 cup almond flour
>
> 1/4 cup sugar
>
> 1 tsp. kosher salt
>
> 6 Tbsp. butter from pastured cows, melted—I use Kerrygold brand

Pat dough into a smooth ball and press into a 9-inch, lightly-greased pie plate. Evenly distribute the dough, pressing it up the sides. Create an edge. I just pressed a fork into mine.

Bake 6-10 minutes at 325 degrees until golden. Remove from oven and cool.

Prepare fresh "jam" by putting the following ingredients into a sauté pan and cook on medium until it comes to a boil, check for sweetness, and take off heat:

> 1 Tbsp. coconut oil
>
> 2 peeled and finely diced peaches
>
> 1 Tbsp. lemon juice
>
> 1 Tbsp. sugar

1 Tbsp. gelatin that is whisked together with 1/4 cup boiling water: NO lumps!

Prepare the filling as follows:

Fill a 3 1/2 quart sauce pan with water and bring to a boil over medium-high heat. Reduce heat to medium to keep at a simmer.

Using an electric mixer with the whisk attachment, whisk the following together in a 2-1/2 quart glass bowl:

3 large eggs

1/3 cup sugar

Place bowl over simmering water and cook while whisking constantly, 5-6 minutes or until mixture becomes slightly thick and sugar dissolves. Remove from heat and the simmering water.

Place 4 tsp. gelatin in a small bowl and pour 1/4 cup boiling water over, whisking constantly until gelatin is completely dissolved.

Using the handheld electric mixer, whisk the egg mixture on high speed for 8-10 minutes until ribbons form on surface of mixture when beater is lifted. Add gelatin mixture and continue whisking one minute more. Fold in the peach "jam" and a pinch of kosher salt.

Spoon filling into cooled pie crust and arrange thin slices of 2 medium peeled peaches over the filling. Cover with plastic wrap and freeze 2 hours.

Serve slices of pie with a dollop of whipped coconut cream sweetened with a pinch of sugar and a splash of vanilla. Going, going, gone!

No Bake Paleo Cobbler with "Benefits"

Certainly berries are powerhouses of antioxidants which fight oxidative stressors that can lead to disease, and they have been shown to sharpen minds and reverse signs of aging, BUT what if we added protein, fiber, collagen, good fats, and anti-inflammatory richness? That's fruit with *benefits*!

Cobbler Topping

In a medium-sized sauté pan on med-low heat, add the following and stir until oils are melted, ingredients are combined, and the mixture becomes browned:

   1 Tbsp. coconut oil

   2 Tbsp. grass fed butter

   1 Tbsp. organic maple syrup, grade B

   1 Tbsp. honey

   1/4 cup ground flax seed

   1/4 cup almond flour

   1 tsp cinnamon

   1/2 cup activated slivered almonds

   1/2 cup unsweetened coconut flakes

Cobbler /or/ Basic Fruit with Benefits (To be eaten alone)

In a large sauté pan on medium-low, add the following:

   2 Tbsp. coconut oil

   3-4 cups of berries and/or fruit cut into small pieces, fresh or frozen

   Dash or two of kosher salt

Generous sprinkling of Ceylon cinnamon

1/4-1/3 cup ground flax seed sprinkled over the fruit

1/4-1/3 cup Great Lakes Gelatin sprinkled over fruit

When fruit begins to bubble and cook in its juices, add:

1 cup water

1 tsp almond extract

Stir occasionally while fruit mixture is gently simmering for 5-10 minutes.

Place fruit mixture into a lightly-oiled, square glass brownie pan or casserole dish of similar size. Spread cobbler topping over the top. Cover and refrigerate or let cool slightly before serving. Garnish with whipped coconut cream, if desired. Great warm, cold, or reheated.

This 'Fruit With Benefits' can also be eaten as-is without the cobbler topping.

Dessert-Like

Chia Seed Smoothies

Just add 2 Tbsp. of chia seeds to your smoothie. If you are stirring, wait at least 15 minutes for the seeds to absorb fluid and stir again. Best if using a high speed blender. They will disappear! Enjoy immediately.

Quick Beneficial Snack

Stir 2 Tbsp. of chia seeds into 1 cup near boiling water. Add 1 Tbsp. of dried fruit or fruit/activated nut blend, add a shake of salt and continue stirring. This will become almost jelly-like, and will hold and satisfy. Great if you need a post-dinner snack!

Anytime Pudding for Breakfast or Dessert

In a blender combine:

1 cup unsweetened coconut /or/ almond milk

1/2 cup plain, unsweetened yogurt, if desired

1-2 dates /or/ 1-2 Tbsp. maple syrup, Grade B

1/2-1 tsp vanilla

Big sprinkle of cinnamon

Pinch of kosher salt

2 Tbsp. or more of chia seeds

1 avocado, peeled and seeded

1/4 cup unsweetened cocoa, if desired

Once you get the hang of this pudding recipe, you will learn it can be tweaked many different ways using different flavorings adding berries, adding fresh mint, no chocolate, no avocado (although it does add smoothness and good fats), more or less milk, more or less yogurt. If you must have a sweeter taste, try some stevia.

Chia Seed and Berry "Jam" or Pudding

In a small pan on medium-low heat, combine:

   1 cup of fresh or frozen blue berries (or other berry)

   1 cup water

   3 Tbsp. chia seeds

   Pinch of salt

   1 teaspoon honey

Optional additions:

   Cinnamon /or/ nutmeg

   Vanilla, almond, /or/ lemon extract

   Lemon zest

Stir occasionally to break up any clumps of seeds and to smash a few of the berries. Bring to bubbling, stir a time or two. That's it! Cooled, it will be almost jam-like and can be used as a spread on gluten-free toast. Dish it up in a bowl. It is a delightful bedtime snack.

Fruit Compote

Ingredients

1-3 Tbsp. coconut oil, depending upon amount of fruit. (I used 3 Tbsp. for a large sauté pan)

1 gala apple, peeled, cored, and chopped into fairly small pieces

1 Bartlett pear, peeled, cored, and chopped into fairly small pieces

2 cups of assorted frozen berries, maybe with some frozen peach

Pinch of salt

Cinnamon to taste, a "sweet spice" that can enhance fruit without the need for sugar. Cinnamon also helps control blood sugar levels

1/4 - 1/3 cup powdered grass-fed gelatin

3 Tbsp. ground flax seed

Optional: One spoonful of honey stirred in at the end only if your fruit is sour

Method

Melt the coconut oil in an enamel, non-stick sauté pan. Add all of the prepared fruit over medium heat. Generously sprinkle the cinnamon, gelatin, and ground flax seed over the top of the fruit. Add a pinch of salt.

As the mixture warms and begins to get juicy, gently stir.

Both the gelatin and the flax will thicken this mixture as the fruit releases its bounteous moisture. If your fruit compote is too runny, just sprinkle on more gelatin and/or more flax. Lower heat a bit to continue cooking without bubbling.

This refrigerates well and can be eaten warm, cold, or at room temperature. So satisfying, filling, good for you, and not sugary!

Main Dishes

Best Ever Salmon Patties

Ingredients

1 (14.75 oz.) can salmon, drained

1 large celery stalk, finely chopped

3-4 green onions, chopped with green stalks

3 mini multi-colored bell peppers, finely chopped

1/2 small can water chestnuts, finely chopped

2-4 eggs, beaten

1 tsp. kosher salt

1 tsp. freshly ground black pepper

1 tsp. dill weed

Approx. 1/4 cup coconut flour, as needed to make the patties "stick" together

Method

Beat eggs in a large bowl.

Add the remaining ingredients, except the coconut flour, and mix well to combine. I do this with my hands while wearing latex-free gloves.

Add the coconut flour if the mixture is too moist (if using 4 eggs) and needs some 'glue' to stick together.

Form mixture into approximately 1/2 cup patties, pressing firmly to mold.

Pan fry the patties on medium heat using about 2 Tbsp. good oil of choice: olive oil, avocado oil, or coconut oil. When the edges start looking a little crispy, flip patties over.

Cooking time should be 2-3 minutes on each side.

Ingredient ideas for dipping sauces:

Using a base of plain Greek yogurt add:

- Dijon mustard, dill weed, lemon zest, lemon juice, pinch of ground red pepper

- Or in a blender or food processor combine the following with the yogurt: English cucumber, dill, salt, and pepper for a Greek flair

Ingredients are easily substituted and swiped out. When there is fresh parsley around, I always add that for added spunk and flakes of greenness. No water chestnuts? Leave them out! I just happened to have a few green onions that needed to be used up; any kind of onion could be used.

Asian Stir Fry

This is what I call a concept recipe. It changes with what is available, but the concept stays the same! Quantities vary according to what's on hand and how many you are serving, as well. There is so much freedom in this kind of recipe!

Prepare all veggies including mincing the garlic ahead of time to allow for a 15-minute resting period, as mentioned in the Foods, Cooking, and Condiments 101 Section.

The Sauce

Assemble and stir up these ingredients in a small bowl for later use:

1-2 cloves garlic, minced

1 inch of fresh ginger, grated /or/ 1 tsp. of powdered ginger

1 small green onion, minced

1/3-1/2 cup of unsweetened pineapple juice from draining one can of unsweetened pineapple chunks or tidbits, which will be used later

1 tsp. of gluten-free fish sauce

1 Tbsp. of coconut aminos /or/ wheat-free Tamari

1 Tbsp. toasted sesame oil

2 Tbsp. of arrowroot

1/2 tsp. crushed red pepper flakes

Stir Fry Veggies and Meat

1/4-1/2 red or yellow onion, chopped into quarter-sized pieces

2 bell peppers (assorted colors, preferable), stemmed and seeded, chopped into quarter-sized pieces

1-2 carrots, peeled and grated

Broccoli florets /or/ other green vegetable such as Bok choy, chopped

Cooked, left-over meat of choice: turkey, chicken, beef, pork, shrimp. Chop or slice thinly based upon meat chosen.

Drained unsweetened pineapple chunks or tidbits

Method

In a fry pan sized to fit the quantity you are cooking, heat 1-2 Tbsp. of ghee, coconut oil, or avocado oil on medium heat setting. Add all vegetables, stir to coat with oil and then stir occasionally. Salt to taste. When onions start to become clear, put a lid on the pan and allow them to steam to a tender-crisp stage.

When vegetables are about done, add drained pineapple and protein of choice. Pour the sauce on top, stir to combine, coat all vegetables and meat. If sauce becomes too thick, add a little bit more of the reserved pineapple juice. When the meat and pineapple are heated, you are ready to eat!

This can be served plain, over zoodles (zucchini noodles), or over white rice if you desire.

Zucchini Pizza Casserole

Our local veggie stand shared a Zucchini Pizza Casserole recipe that I have used as a casserole and as a pizza-on-the-stone crust. This recipe does call for cheese; but for me, it is a worthy treat!

Ingredients

4 cups unpeeled zucchini noodles (can also be done with a cheese shredder)

1/2 teaspoon salt

2 eggs

1/2 cup grated Parmesan cheese

2 cups mozzarella cheese, divided

1 cup shredded cheddar cheese, divided

1 lb. ground beef

1/2 cup chopped onion

1 medium bell pepper, chopped

Homemade Sauce

1 clove garlic, minced

1 small can tomato paste with one-two cans water

1 teaspoon fish sauce

Salt

Pepper

Pinch of sugar

Italian Seasoning to taste

1/4 teaspoon anise seed

Sauté garlic in ghee 30 seconds, add other ingredients, stir to combine, simmer to meld flavors.

Grate or spiralize the zucchini into noodles. Place zucchini in strainer and sprinkle with salt. Let stand at least 10 minutes. Sprinkle zucchini over a clean towel, roll up, and gently squeeze out the moisture.

Combine zucchini with eggs, Parmesan, and half of the mozzarella and cheddar cheeses. Press mixture into a greased 13 x 9 inch baking dish.

Bake uncovered at 400 degrees for 20 minutes.

Meanwhile, cook beef and onion over medium heat until meat is no longer pink. Drain. Add tomato sauce, spoon over baked zucchini. Sprinkle with remaining cheeses. Add bell pepper.

Bake 20 minutes longer until heated through.

Pizza Crust the Second Way

My all-time favorite bread-y pizza dough recipe is on the glutenfreegoddess.com website. There are many different gluten-free flours used, so when I gather all of the ingredients, I create three extra containers of dry ingredients. It's so nice to grab my homemade "mix" and just add the wet ingredients and the yeast so we can have pizza on the spur of the moment!

Extras

Cashew Gravy

Great on all kinds of meat. Freezes and reheats well. This is a go-to gravy indeed!

Ingredients

3 large onions, diced

3/4 cup cashew butter (I make my own by processing cashews a very long time in the food processor; eventually the butter will form)

1/3 cup tamari, make sure it is gluten-free (it's like soy sauce)

3 Tbsp. extra virgin olive oil

1/4 tsp. pepper

1/4 tsp. sage

2-1/2 cup water

Method

Using a large bottomed skillet over medium heat, sauté the onions for a long time—probably 20 minutes,—until they caramelize. Not much stirring is needed early on in the process, but as they become more cooked, more frequent attention is needed.

Once the onions are starting to turn golden, add the water, cashew butter, tamari, pepper, and sage.

Add the cashew butter to the onions, stir to incorporate, and allow them to cook a few minutes. Process in about three batches in the food processor or blender, blitzing until smooth. Pour the gravy into a sauce pan to finish cooking a bit. Use what you need, freeze the rest, and you will be in gravy for a while.

Sweet Basil Pesto

Pesto can be a great spread on crackers, bread, or as a great way to zip up the flavor factor in veggies, sea food, or an omelet.

Ingredients

2 cups fresh sweet basil leaves, packed

1/2 cup Parmesan, Parmesan-Reggiano, /or/ Romano cheese, grated

1/2 cup extra virgin olive oil

1/3 cup walnuts /or/ pine nuts (activate nuts first!)

3 cloves garlic

Salt and fresh ground pepper to taste (I used not quite a ½ tsp. of kosher salt and about the same of black pepper)

Method

Using a food processor, pulse the nuts a few times. Add the garlic cloves and pulse some more. Add the basil and pulse until in fine pieces. With the food processor fully on, slowly pour the olive oil through the shoot. Stop to scrape the sides down and add the grated cheese. Pulse until combined. Add salt and pepper and pulse a few more times.

The pesto is ready to use. I store mine in small jars and float additional olive oil on top as a seal.

Activated Nuts

Raw nuts are better than nuts highly processed in 'Franken oils,' but raw nuts still have factors in them that inhibit proper absorption and can contribute to unhappy tummies. Enter the "activated nut," which has been handled in such a way as to eliminate the anti-digestive phytates and to activate beneficial digestive enzymes instead.

Activated nuts require soaking, at least; and dehydrating for long-term storage.

To Soak

Using glass bowls (I have learned nuts will actually permanently discolor metal bowls!), dissolve about 1 tsp. of sea salt in 6 cups water, add raw nuts, and soak. I buy large bags of nuts, so this requires multiple bowls. Walnuts, almonds, and pecans can soak 12 hours; cashews take just 6 hours. The water will turn quite brown.

Thoroughly rinse soaked nuts, and spread out on towels (I have a bath towel dedicated to this process—some staining may occur). Roll the towel up and let the towel soak up any extra moisture for a few minutes. If nuts will be used in a blender or food processor, they may be used now; but if long-term storage is desired, dehydrating is necessary.

To Dehydrate

If using a dehydrator, spread nuts out in a single layer on each tray needed, allowing for a good circulation of air around the nuts. Do not crowd them. Place trays in the dehydrator. Set temperature for 115-125 degrees and set for 12 hours. Check for dryness when time is up. Lengthen that time as needed. Store in a closed container in a cool environment.

If using the oven method, spread the nuts out on large baking trays. Do not crowd them. Set oven for lowest temperature possible. Since oven heat will be higher than the dehydrator, the drying time will be shorter. Stir the nuts every hour and check on crispness after 6 hours. Store in a closed container in a cool environment.

Trail Mix

    2 cups walnuts

    2 cups pecans

    2 cups unsweetened coconut chips (large flakes)

    1/2 cup dried blueberries

    1/2 cup dried cherries

    1/3 cup mini dark chocolate morsels

Just mix, put into handy baggies, and enjoy where ever you go!

Date Jewels

A great appetizer or special taste treat to any meal, these take very little time to prepare and are easily reheated in a toaster oven.

Dates, seeds removed

Nitrate-free bacon

Ground pork sausage OR goat cheese

Soak dates for 15-30 minutes in hot water to soften; drain dates. Put about a teaspoonful of sausage meat OR goat cheese inside dates. Wrap each date with 1/3 - 1/2 slice of bacon; place wrapped date on a foil-covered oven-safe pan with the seam side of the overlapping bacon on the pan side. Bake uncovered for 30 minutes at 350 degrees. These are exceedingly hot due to the natural sugar in the dates, so let cool a few minutes.

Gluten-free, Dairy-free, Savory and Cheesy Kale Chips

Soak ¾ cup (preferably raw, unprocessed) cashews in water for at least one hour.

Assemble the following ingredients and put into a food processor:

  1 large clove of garlic, peeled and sliced

  2 Tbsp. coconut aminos (a gluten-free version of soy sauce /or/ you can use wheat-free tamari)

  2 Tbsp. avocado oil /or/ coconut oil

  1/3 cup nutritional yeast

  1 lemon, juiced

  1/8 tsp. smoked paprika

  1/8 tsp. salt

Process soaked, drained cashews and the ingredients listed in a food processor until a smooth paste is formed.

Prepare kales leaves by thoroughly washing, drying, and removing the main stem and pulling off any firmer 'arteries' that come off of the main stem.

Evenly distribute paste over one bunch of cleaned and prepped kale leaves. Massage leaves with paste to work in the goodness and to break down the kale a bit. This should take about 5 minutes to accomplish.

Evenly space prepared chips onto parchment-covered baking sheets. Bake in 180 degree oven for 1 hour; turn leaves over; continue baking about 45-60 more minutes until all leaves are crispy. Store in a zip lock bag. Enjoy!

SPECIAL TIMES

It's actually getting easier to successfully stay on the 80 side of 80/20 while dining out. My favorite breakfast stop is a bagel shop! I just do not eat the bagels. There is always some interesting egg scramble or omelet they are whipping up that more than satisfies! Their chicken salad on a salad is awesome—just hold the croutons.

Just about every restaurant has a gluten-free menu. Substitutions for a second vegetable instead of a baked potato are easily honored. Instead of breaded and fried seafood, broiled or pan fried has never been a problem to get.

If you have severe food allergies, it is a necessity to understand the menu. Asking to speak with the chef is the best way to make sure there are no ingredients that contain wheat or other harm-causing factors. People who create meals for others want to please.

Mostly for the rest of us, it's a matter of choice. Choose to honor your body and all of the good you have accomplished with it.

Holidays and special events are scattered around the calendar and are numerous enough to actually 'hold hands' with each other throughout the year. Throwing caution to the wind for special occasions could easily mean you no longer care about supporting your body's health. In other words, those looking for an 'excuse' do not have far to look.

Clear heads, glowing skin, happy bellies, trimmer waists, rock solid blood sugars, body joints that no longer swell and hurt—gosh! Do you really want to give those many good things up?

Celebrations are about good company, laughing, and sharing! They can all be accomplished while eating an anti-inflammatory diet.

While you are with a group, go ahead, make that birthday cake! Even Betty Crocker has a box for that (with additives, though). Make your own buttercream icing—without the chemicals—or frost it using whipped coconut cream to lessen the sugar hit. Enjoy! Blow out the candles! Share with everyone why you look and feel so good!

Thanksgiving Notes

Feast Days do not have to ruin the good balance we have achieved in eating for good health. Take note of the following ideas as you begin to plan for Thanksgiving or other holiday meals.

Turkey: Of course, if feasible, free-range would be a plus; but otherwise, make sure there are giblets with the bird. Use the neck, heart, and gizzard as a base for the gravy. Place them in a large sauce pan with water, chunks of one onion, and several ribs of celery along with salt, pepper, and poultry seasoning for a several-hour simmer. Take out the giblets, remove and finely chop the meat. Return meat to the pot, raise the heat to a gentle boil, and stir in 2-3 Tbsp. of arrowroot dissolved in ¼ cup water to thicken the gravy, lower the heat and let it reduce. Gently sauté the liver in ghee, with salt and pepper; mash with a fork and a spoonful of mayo /or/ yogurt along with your favorite herb for a quick pate to enjoy while waiting on the "bird" to finish cooking.

Ham: There exists ham that is gluten-free. Apparently, gluten is often used in the processing of ham, so those with serious gluten concerns, beware. I know Sam's carries gluten-free ham; but always watch out for that packet of glaze. Geez! So many ingredients......and probably wheat starch to boot, along with the high-fructose corn syrup solids. Stick with a homemade glaze of honey and mustard.

Cranberries: You can use half the sugar and never miss it if you just add the juice of one large orange. I have also come to love adding one diced pear, one diced apple, and a handful of raspberries to the mixture. Awesome! If you use that much fruit, you can cut the water down, too.

Dressing: Yes, it can be gluten-free. Use part of a recipe of Bob's Red Mill gluten-free corn bread mix package, let it dry out overnight along with a few slices of gluten-free bread (from the freezer section of the grocery store) that has also dried out. Dice up the dried breads and place into a large bowl. Once you have sautéed one diced onion and about 3 ribs of celery in some Kerrygold butter and poultry seasoning, add ¾ cup broth or water and pour over breads mixture. Toss to combine and place into a buttered baking dish. Bake, covered, in a 350 degree oven for 30 minutes. This may be gluten-free, but this is a starch, so invite a lot of people so the leftovers won't tempt you too badly.

Roasted root vegetables can be a feast in and of themselves. They are certainly better for us than Aunt Jean's Sweet Potato Fluff, which is sweet enough to be a dessert! The smell of root vegetables tossed with olive oil and fresh spices such as rosemary and thyme will set everyone's mouth to watering.

Green Veggies: Repeat after me, "Veggies do not require a can of creamed soup!" Enjoy nature's bounty by lightly sautéing veggies in ghee or olive oil, steaming with 1-2 Tbsp. of water to complete cooking, and possibly finish with a splash of toasted sesame oil.

Pumpkin Pie: My favorite can actually be enjoyed without a pie crust, although gluten-free crust mixes are out there. Try baking your pie with reduced sugar. Try making a meringue out of the egg whites first and then fold in the rest of the ingredients. Using a meringue as a base makes baking it without a crust very easy. To make this non-dairy, simply reduce your favorite non-dairy milk over a medium heat, stirring constantly, to create condensed milk. It should reduce by 50% (2 cups become 1 cup). I love healthy pumpkin fluff!

Mince Meat Pie: An old favorite from when I was growing up, but now I use ½ of a jar of mince meat mixture to flavor about three chopped up apples that have been tossed in 23 Tbsp. of arrowroot as thickening. A lower-sugar alternative and a great way to have apple pie, too.

Once you get into the swing of recipe modification, having celebratory foods that support a healthy body are not so hard to do. The Internet is full of anti-inflammatory/Paleo recipes of every type.

Well, isn't it interesting that Chapter Thirteen is about exercise?! That's what's next! Lucky thirteen!

EXERCISES

NOTE: For your safety: please work with your doctor or physical therapist before starting any kind of exercise routine! Each one of us has specific needs and limitations that need to be recognized and met. If any exercise does not feel "right" while you are doing it, then STOP. If balance is an issue, always make sure you have something secure to hold on to. Safety first in all things!

Studying about habits, positive outlooks, whole foods, paleo, the ravages of gluten, and recipes that fit into real life, is where my passion is.

I am much less experienced in exercise, however; and improving my own health and exercise status is an on-going thing. But there's great news! I have picked up some tips and pointers that not only made sense on paper, but have fleshed out in real progress for myself. My whole approach to exercise has shifted to a totally positive, excited anticipation of what I will be doing each day.

When first starting to write this book in February of 2015, I followed my own advice and started to chip away at this exercise "thing" by taking tiny steps. I have shared with you throughout this book the gradual, steady success I was achieving with my planks.

My approach to doing planks started with a cerebral understanding of how habits worked and how to grow them through consistent application of daily small efforts. I checked off on my Easy Tweaks Habit Tracker the planks (always) and other short exercises (usually) I did each day. As described throughout this book, I could see my strength and endurance increase over time, and that felt so good!

But I had not yet crossed over into a joyous embrace of what I was doing. I did not understand the power of combining this exercise routine into something greater. I named what I called an "ideal" morning routine a "Series of Good Things." This series started with that extra glass of water first thing in the morning and morphed into mindful breathing, prayer, reading the Bible, and finishing by doing exercise "while the coffee/tea was brewing."

But it was still something of a cerebral thing. I described earlier in this book I had not made the commitment to giving this special time any kind of priority. If it happened in the morning, great. If it didn't happen first thing in the morning and had to be done later in the day, that was okay, too. Maybe tomorrow I would "happen" upon a great morning. It was a choice on my part.

That is, until my whole mindset changed by reading, *The Miracle Morning* by Hal Elrod. He brought the enthusiasm and heart into my "Series of Good Things." His shares his personal story of overcoming significant disability by focusing on his morning routine. Not only did he overcome his disabilities, but he soared to record-breaking heights in the business world by doing and living his Miracle Morning!

It's August 2015 now, and I am putting the final touches on *Toolkit for Wellness*. In less than 30 days since reading his book, I have totally embraced my own "Series of Good Things" by prioritizing them. Thank you, Hal! I anticipate each night what I am going to do the next morning upon rising. The big switch for me is that I AM GETTING UP EARLIER to do this each day!

I share this with you, dear reader, to point out that we are all works in progress. We are all on a journey. Even in the course of writing this book for you, I have grown in the steady application of what I am sharing with you AND in what I am learning, even up to the time of publication!

You can do this, too! That's the message!

A real walk along the path of mind-body-spirit wellness is incomplete without exercise. Even the ancient philosophers touted the importance of physical exercise to balance the exercise of expanding and training our minds.

Everything we need to do in terms of meaningful exercise can be done at home; gym membership is not essential unless you are seriously into cross-fit or training for a major sports event. Many Paleo enthusiasts summarize exercise into moving around a lot (walking mostly and jog/run a bit) and lifting heavy things (wisely, be safe at all times).

A Big Little Secret About Exercise!

One thing that had held me back with exercise was, after finally mastering an exercise, I was rewarded with the opportunity... to do *more*! This seemed to be a poor reward and a potential time drain to me! Walk or jog a mile. Then two. Then ten....gee! Where does this stop, you know? I did not want to sign up for that; but I *did* want to maintain or increase my muscle tone, strength, and range of motion.

What to do? Then I learned about the science of movement that solved my dilemmas, erased my excuses, and gave me hope.

I have learned from reading and listening to the experts that simply increasing the number of repetitions in an exercise, say squats, is not going to exercise the right kinds of muscle fibers for maximum benefit (getting in shape and burning fat, baby!). What is needed is an increase in the *load* we are bearing when doing that movement. This can be accomplished in two ways:

1. Add weight we are holding, and/or

2. Slowing down the movement into a slow motion effort

Personally, I just love this! I am not inclined to be spending a longer period of time exercising (doing more repetitions). If I am easily nailing squats, then slowing them down increases the work load dramatically. By slow I mean, squat down to a count of 10, hold for 10, and slowly rise to a count of 10.

Doing slow-motion exercises actually results in doing *fewer* repetitions because the workload is so much greater. Once five slow-motion squats are easy, then ramp up the workload by adding small weights to your hands. Then, increase the weight over time to increase your effort. It works!

Not ready for push-ups? Start with kitchen counter push-ups. Placing hands on the counter top edge, step back two or three feet and commence to doing push-ups. They are quite easy, and I have to warn you, it would be easy to do twenty; but the next day, you'll know you have overdone it.

If you think you have the kitchen counter push-ups knocked, next try slowing them down. Slow means counting to 10 on the way down, holding for 10, and slowly rising for a count of 10. Whew! If you can do 5 of those in slow motion, you are ready to increase the work load by finding a lower hand hold such as on a non-movable bench.

Mastered those? The floor is next. Regular speed push-ups first. Then, rather than doing 100 of them, do just a few very slowly. Saves time and really works the part of the muscle that burns fat!

Planks

Remember my story about learning to do planks? Start with tiny goals. It's amazing how muscles quickly grow accustomed to working when the job is broken down into small parts. In fact, it is now August 2015. My plank experience has grown from half-planks to full planks, to...oh, I am so tickled to say this: PUSH-UPS! Me! I had NEVER done pushups before! This Grandma is doing them! You can, too!

To refresh the method: Planks are done by lying down facing the floor. Raise your body up, resting weight just on elbows/forearms and toes. Your body should be in a straight line. A half-plank would have you resting your weight on elbows/forearms and knees.

I've even improved upon the timing method for doing my 1 minute plank. Staring at my watch was boring and a bit defeatist. Can I last 15 more seconds? And, did I say it was boring? A switch to counting down deep-breathing was much more effective for me. It takes me 12 slow, long deep breaths to do a minute plank and the results are so much better. One point of exercise is to get the life-giving oxygen all around the body, so this just helps that goal. And it is not boring.

Push-Ups

The story of the push-ups will sound familiar. After knocking out my "12 breaths" planks, I started with half-body push-ups. They were okay push-ups...not deep ones, but I angled and straightened my arms 5 times. Then 10 times. Then 10 deeper push-ups.

Then I would precede those 10 half-push-ups with 5 not-so-great full body push-ups. You know the kind: barely angle the arm and straighten back up? But, hey! It was a start and I KNEW I was on my way.

Today, I am improving the form and quality of my full and half-body push-ups each day!

Just do it EVERY DAY!

The Slant

Another short, easy exercise is the slant. Great for thighs, "buns of steel," and the core; the time slanting can be gradually increased as well. To do a slant, lie on your back with knees bent, feet on the ground. Lift your buttocks up until your trunk and thighs are in a straight line. Hold for as long as you want. If you can easily do this for one minute, try adding a weight to your belly... a book, a toddler... just be safe and gradually increase your load.

Ten to fifteen minutes is about my limit for serious exercise, and it is really sweet to know I can work my whole body with just a few repetitions of a few exercises.

Practice Balancing EVERY Day!

Maintaining balance is ever so important, too. I know of people who lose their balance while standing still, let alone when in motion.

Not only is this a safety thing, but a mobility thing. Staying mobile under our own steam, so-to-speak, is of paramount importance. Practice should start early in life. As always—it's never too late to start.

Keeping in mind, habit stacking makes doing new things easier! Here are two suggestions for simple balance exercises.

One of my *Designed for Health* students shared with the class that he and his wife always made it a habit to stand on one foot or the other whenever waiting in line at the grocery store. The grocery basket was there to touch or hold for balance checks, and they were doing something productive while waiting in line.

Our daughter said she always practices standing on one foot then the other while brushing her teeth. You know how electric toothbrushes are set for two minutes? That's one minute on one foot while brushing the bottom teeth, and another minute on the other foot while brushing the top teeth. You have already committed two minutes to something else so why not "tweak" that time by "habit stacking" to improve your balance? Make sure you have one free hand to touch or hold on to the counter for any balance checks or increased stability needs. Always be safe!

So, join me in looking like a flamingo while brushing your teeth or waiting in line! It's fun!

Getting the Heart Rate Up

This is the part I do while the coffee or tea is brewing each morning and it is my favorite.

This simple exercise hits on so many things: Getting the heart rate up, pumping oxygen all around to get my brain in high gear, improving balance, range of motion, endurance, and joint health.

This routine can last as long as you wish. I have so much fun doing it, some days the winding down lasts a little longer because I like the "rush."

I start by taking slow, high-steps while standing in place, raising my knee as high as I can. This is another balance thing, so always make sure there is a counter or chair back to touch or hold on to for balance checks. My balance is good, so sometimes I will slowly prance around the living room. I might take 20 high steps, but 10 would do nicely.

Next, the tempo increases slightly and the knees do not come up as far. Listen to the beat of your steps. By now, I am taking these steps in place. This is done for 10-20 more steps.

Gradually, the pace picks up again and again. Ladies: Somewhere in here I hold my chest so my breasts don't bounce! These exercises do not require changing into a sports bra for so little an investment in time. Just "hold 'em!"

At peak speed, my goal is to be like those football players in training where they run at their fastest pace while standing in place. I do not stay at the peak speed for long. It just depends on what I feel like doing.

The rest of this awesome blood pumping exercise is a gradual reversing of the process. Listening for the tempo, gradually ramp down the speed of your steps and increase the height of your knees until you return to the leisurely "prance" of stepping high.

By the end of this exercise, you will be wanting to tackle the day's projects!

Fly Like an Eagle!

While your legs are cooling off from that stationary "run," give your arms a simple workout. I learned the palms-up method from Teresa Tapp in her TTapp exercises available online for purchase.

When we think of doing arm circles, we usually do them with our palms facing the floor. But when doing any kind of straight arm exercises, turning the palms to face the ceiling totally changes the muscle dynamics.

Standing "at ease" with feet shoulder-width apart, knees slightly bent, and pelvis tucked, hold your arms straight out to your side. Reach out hard like you are trying to touch the walls. You are now making a "T" shape. Here's the difference. Keep the palms of your hands facing the ceiling.

Now, at a moderate pace, drop your straight arms down toward your side about one third of the way down and back up 8 times. Easy enough. Next, drop them two thirds of the way down and back up 8 times. Okay... Next drop them down all the way and back up 8 times. Whoa!

That was a totally different dynamic, wasn't it? If you can still keep those arms up with palms still facing the ceiling, do 20 arm circles forward followed by 20 arm circles going backward.

Still up for some more? Finish by pulsing those straight arms back about 20 times.

Excellent!

In Motion with Nature

Needless to say, walking remains a keystone to any exercise routine. Whether you intentionally walk around the neighborhood or go someplace special to walk, it's all good. Walking can certainly be incorporated (habit-stacked) into our daily errands just by parking farther from the stores and parking at the farthest end of the mall from where we are going. Why wait for after work? Take just 10 minutes of your lunch to walk outside for a double benefit of stress relief:

exercise coupled with the mental stress release of being outside in the open air!

It's no accident dog owners have a healthy edge. They are outdoors walking Fido at least twice a day. Plus there is all of that unconditional love! A winning combination for those who can.

Meditative Exercise!

Active exercise is a great way to decrease stress in addition to its other body-toning and oxygenation benefits. But that's just part of the picture.

One of the best tools in your *Toolkit for Wellness* is yoga! Yoga had always been something I was going to 'get around to' someday. Naturally, that was a choice to not do it.

It's all about choice and in choosing to put our own health first. How can we be of any benefit to helping others if we are falling apart? Remember what they say on airplanes? "Put on your own oxygen mask *first* before even helping the child next to you." We have to keep our own Self balanced!

Yoga is just so healing, nurturing, and safe feeling. It has been a real game-changer for me. As a caregiver with ever-increasing responsibilities, feeling overwhelmed is a common occurrence. To keep things in perspective, to stop the merry-go-round, and to regain composure and inner flow, yoga has been key.

The weekly class I attend is a Yin Yoga class. We do not balance in Warrior poses! All of what we do is from the floor while on our mats. It is a practice not of movement or strength, but a practice of allowing and opening. The mindful process of poses is gentle and allowing, never strained or stressed.

Our bodies' natural flow of energies are opened up. It is detoxifying and releasing in both a spiritual and a physical way. We release pent-up toxic energies from our minds and spirits by being mindful of our breathing. Aside from feeling clearer, cleaner, and lighter, the proof of toxin release from our bodies comes if we forget to drink extra water to help flush them out. A general malaise will wash over you if you do not help the toxin's permanent 'exit' from your body with extra hydration!

In addition to the tools of daily mindful breathing, meditation, and prayer, time spent in yoga grounds and stabilizes both mentally and physically. Do not miss using this tool!

Take Away Thoughts:

- Like the Starter Recipe Chapter, this is not intended to be an end-all, do-all exercise resource. Instead, I hoped to share with you some basic things you can do at home within your regular routine that would substantially help with your over-all muscle tone and balance.

- It was liberating to me to learn the muscle fibers that burn fat and rev-up metabolism are *not* the ones addressed in endurance training! Strength training by increasing the "load" factor in muscle movement is a very agreeable and user friendly approach to short, yet complete, workouts.

Take Away Actions:

- Put the joy into your "Series of Good Things" by checking out Hal Elrod's book, *Miracle Morning*.

- Liberate your energies by doing your own "Series of Good Things" first thing in the morning. Getting up earlier never felt so good! Try it for a week before you fall back saying, "I'm not a morning person!" My personal productivity has drastically increased because of it! I wasn't a morning person either.

- Set your exercise goals very small. Start working towards a one minute (half) plank if you wish. Add a slant. Add a push-up.

- Habit-stack exercise time. What about "while the coffee is brewing"? A limited commitment and very doable.

- Do a few squats, a few (kitchen counter) push-ups, a round of running in place, and "flap your wings palms up".

- Increase the load of your movements by adding weight and/or by slowing down the motions.

- Just do it! Every day!

It's sort of sad to think this is nearing the end of 'our' book! Thanks for checking it out! My goal is to help you in some small way help clear the confusion about what is healthy, to give you the tools and the power of understanding, and to guide you through successful change, which will be fulfilled as you take ACTION in your daily life to help yourself. There is just one more bit of advice I need to share with you, so please keep reading.

HAVE FUN, NOT ULCERS!

It's been a long journey, this wellness thing. Recognizing that our mind, body, and spirit should be in lock-step is no small matter. Accepting responsibility for your smooth, harmonious functioning should feel more and more natural as you practice what you have learned.

Everything within us, and about us, is so interconnected. Becoming an informed, mindful, active partner with your body is a life-long journey. Once the understanding of your own inner connectedness is established, respected, and honored, you can benefit from heights of wellness you never thought possible!

This *Toolkit for Wellness* was designed to empower you. Knowledge *is* power because truly *learning* something results in a change of behavior. You have discovered the tools to better control your wellness destiny by learning about simple, doable, and repeatable tweaks. These "tweaks," or steps you take, will promote you to a higher level of wellness immediately.

You have learned being proactive for your health is a daily choice. No one else can do it for you. We cannot just be swept along with the tide of what "everybody is doing." Just looking around us will demonstrate that approach does not work. There are economic forces creating a lot of misinformation. You now have the tools to understand the difference in what you see and hear.

Learning about how your digestive system works should be arming you to make choices to defend it. Understanding the anti-inflammatory diet should be opening your eyes to past causes of dis-ease and how to promote your gut healing today and in the future.

You have learned high levels of stress are not just something we need to "man-up" to. Stress is more than just a load on our nerves; it's a load on every body system. Stress and sleep-deprived nights can derail our hunger hormones and our ability to process blood sugars. No wonder we have the saying, "Stress kills!"

You are armed with a deeper understanding of how habits work. You know how to use that knowledge to make small changes over time to create great progress and change. An "easy tweaks" approach is an arsenal of tools you can use to conquer changing habits without relying on waning willpower stores.

You have a whole list of tools to use to restore your sleep. Motivation to improve your sleep has increased and has become urgent since you learned how a restful night sets you up for balanced hormones for hunger and carbohydrate processing.

You have the key tools to balance blood sugars and you understand how to "measure" what is good for you to eat.

The power of inflammation and the destruction it leaves in its wake has been a wake-up call for immediate action. Best of all, you have the tools at your fingertips to stop inflammation and begin the healing right now. Starter recipes and several key "secrets" are enabling you to heal your body with every meal.

A "Series of Good Things" includes easy, repeatable exercises that can grow in intensity, yet not consume your day. You have followed this Grandma as she journeyed through planks and push-ups to learn that you can do it, too! It is never too late to start a program of self-improvement and renewal!

We are *designed for health*! The dis-ease and diseases that are flooding our nation and wherever the Western lifestyle is embraced are not natural. In the scheme of things, we are headed for total physical destruction. Over time, we should be *increasing* our life span, not shortening it. Children today have shorter projected lifespans than their parents! Why are we seeing such a wave of diabetes, obesity, and auto-immune diseases? You now know part of the answer. What we have been eating has not complimented our natural processes.

You have been given the tools of understanding and empowerment to immediately see benefits from the small changes recommended here that will increase your wellness. You know how to use them!

Using these tools should be easy! Life is meant to be enjoyed! I want you to enjoy your days **more** by feeling better, more balanced, and not weighted-down with disease. This is a **good** thing!

We have to create a natural, doable, daily flow without any sense of restriction. It's all in our point of view. Case in point: I have always felt being married is liberating. Many people regard marriage as being tied down and restricted to just one partner. On the contrary! For us, being married set us both free to fully love each other. To have a partner forever to explore and experience life together. To always have someone's back. It's a *good* thing!

Discovering what works, is synchronous, and naturally beneficial and healing for our bodies can only be liberating! How can choosing feeling vibrant, energized, and balanced be a bad thing?

Consider your approach. For example, even as a marginal soda drinker, I still went through a gradual paring down of how much I drank soda until I just stopped. Do I sit hang-faced and grumpy around others who drink it? Do I look superior and tell others they shouldn't be drinking it? Additionally, do I stress about hidden sugar in a splash of restaurant salad dressing? I hope not!

We can cheerfully share with others what we do and why we do it when the opportunity is right. There is a lot of good wellness information to share indeed. Just remember to go easy on yourself and others. It's 80/20, remember? Converting to an anti-inflammatory life style should be easy and natural, not obsessive or restrictive.

We need to loosen up! At the same time, we should joyfully embrace all we know about what is going to "do our body good."

Have fun, not ulcers!

RESOURCES

A peek at the book shelf:

The Paleo Solution, Robb Wolf

Primal Blueprint, Mark Sisson

The Calorie Myth, Jonathan Bailor

Your Personal Paleo Code, Chris Kresser

10-Day Detox Diet, Mark Hyman, MD

Death By Food Pyramid, Denise Minger

Against All Grain, Danielle Walker

Eat Like a Dinosaur, The Paleo Parents

Nom Nom Paleo, Michelle Tam and Henry Fong

The Micro-nutrient Miracle, Jayson Calton, PhD and Mira Calton, CN

The Miracle Morning, Hal Elrod

Never Too Late: Your Roadmap to Reinvention, Claire Cook

The 18 Rules of Happiness, Karl Moore

The Art of Persistence, Michal Stawicki

Trickle Down Mindset, Michal Stawicki

The Slight Edge, Jeff Olson

Book Launch, Chandler Bolt

Important resource for Multiple Sclerosis patients:

The Wahls Protocol: How I Beat Progressive MS Using Paleo Principles and

Functional Medicine, Terry Wahls, MD

Subscribing:

Foodtalk4you.com

Jamesclear.com

Marksdailyapple.com

Paleohacks.com

SCDlifestyle.com

Thedr.com

Chriskresser.com

SummerBock.com

SaraGottfriedMD.com

Jonathan Bailor at sanesolution.com

Alexandra Jamieson

Where to get gluten free, paleo, vegan, dairy free foods, condiments, nuts, seeds, oils, and a lot of other healthful stuff mentioned in this book: Thrivemarket.com

In addition to Thrive Market's site above, for all things coconut I also use: Tropical Traditions

Where to get grass fed meats and fresh caught fish and seafood: US Wellness Meats

THANK YOU

Creating this book has been a gift to *you*. Along with every word typed was the hope that some thought shared here would resonate with you, give you an "ah-ha" moment, and set you fully equipped with the tools to start on your journey of easy, naturally obtained, wellness.

Please take a moment to leave an honest review on Amazon and share with others how Toolkit for Wellness has helped you.

ACKNOWLEDGMENTS

I thank God for bringing me to this point; equipping me and surrounding me with a steady flow of the right people who have provided the continued inspiration, knowledge, and support to keep me going and energized!

My family's support and guidance has been crucial. Thank you to my husband, Virgil, who always made sure I was properly equipped both in the kitchen 'laboratory' and in the office. His support of my 'holing up' in the office to write has been unwavering. Our son, James, rescued me more than once on FaceTime from hardware and software Mommy Meltdown Moments. His easy comfort in experimenting with blending flavors has expanded my approach to seasoning and meal enhancement. Our daughter, Serena, opened the Paleo door to our mutual interest in better eating which was critical to my research. Her naturally mindful approach to life, food, and creative cooking continues to inspire and lead me to a proper balance in all things. Cooking alongside our children is always the best of experiences. Our daughter-in-law, Amy, shared so many new ideas with me about cooking, flavors, and the wonders of vegetables at breakfast. Katie and Sam, our grandchildren, continue to be shining examples of how clean eating can boost growth and development in young minds and bodies.

Thanks to Donna Stortz, my co-teacher at West Craven High School, who was a co-researcher and experimenter in all things Paleo while we were working together, and who provided the initial encouragement to write this book. Sheree Alderman, my right hand lady, is not only a personal cheerleader but has enabled my website to be beautiful! Her inspiration as a writer herself catapulted my efforts to spread my message through the written word. Thank you for being my friend and editor. Anna Pearson: special thanks for being my beta reader and for catching many mistakes before I pressed 'publish'. Anthony Smits, your insight and ideas have been invaluable.

Dr. Sharon Bender at First Baptist Church, New Bern, North Carolina, thank you for encouraging me to lead the first Designed for Health classes at church. The interest, excitement, and the openness to learning about wellness from the Designed for Health students provided even more motivation for me to spread the word. My heart-felt thanks!

Robert Cheung and Elizabeth Brinkley—thank you for sharing your personal triumphs with me and encouraging me. Ellen Sink; you are an amazing Yoga teacher.

To other people who inspire their own readers with understanding about habits, perseverance, personal growth— you will never know the depth of how your words moved me from an idea to an action. Thank you: James Clear, Alexandra Jamieson, Michal Stawicki, Karl Moore, Claire Cook, Jeff Goins, and Jeff Olsen.

Lastly, special thanks to Chandler Bolt whose guidance through his Book Launch series and especially his Self-Publishing School have enabled me to go from good to awesome, from writing to actual publishing. SPS has provided the roadmap and the guide to what I needed to do, step by step. My coach, Hahna Kane Latonick, has been there to listen, guide, and offer suggestions and understanding at all times. To our SPS Mastermind Community and my Accountability Partner,

Marilyn Betlach, you are the best for ideas, support, in depth opinion polls, and encouragement throughout this amazing process in self growth! Friends at the *Positively Perfect* Launch Team, what an awesome, helpful group!

Toolkit for Wellness Launch Team, you rock! Thanks!

ABOUT THE AUTHOR

Deidre Edwards knows from experience that it is never too late for self-growth and transformation. Finding yet another avenue to share her medical background, teaching skills, and passion for self-improvement and natural healing, she is now sharing with others her discoveries to total mind-body-spirit wellness through her writing and Designed for Health Seminars.

Her daughter's decade-long struggle with undiagnosed Celiac Disease initially drove her to seek answers beyond conventional wisdom, and Deidre dived into a deeper study of how foods affect the body, mind, and spirit. She discovered that there was much more to the story than what the Food Pyramid and the 'whole grain goodness' movements were saying.

After nearly 20 years as a Registered Nurse and National Board Certified Teacher in Career and Technical Education/Health Sciences, Deidre is taking her talent for breaking down information into understandable parts and sharing what she has learned with adult audiences of every age.

Deidre is a firm believer that we were designed for health and not disease, and she enjoys shining a light on how to use food, mindfulness, and exercise for the good of our bodies. It thrills her to see others reverse many of their conditions by putting into practice the simple concepts that she teaches.

Disclaimer: Deidre would like to remind her informed readers that she is a sharer of information, not a medical expert. All readers should rely on the advice of their health care providers when implementing any dietary or exercise changes.

For comments or to book a Designed for Health Seminar, contact Deidre on her website at www.foodtalk4you.com or email her at foodtalk4you@gmail.com.